NATURE'S GIFT OF FOOD

With my
best wishes.

Jan de Vries

Nature's Gift series

FOOD

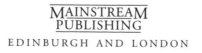

MAINSTREAM
PUBLISHING
EDINBURGH AND LONDON

This edition 2005

Copyright © Jan de Vries, 1992

First published in Great Britain in 1992 by
MAINSTREAM PUBLISHING COMPANY (EDINBURGH) LTD
7 Albany Street
Edinburgh EH1 3UG

ISBN 1 84018 628 3

A catalogue record for this book is available from the British Library

Typeset in Garamond
Printed and bound in Great Britain by
Antony Rowe Ltd, Chippenham, Wiltshire

Truth, Power, Beauty lie in Simplicity.
(saying by Tagore)

Contents

1

Healthy Eating

ONE MORNING, FULL of enthusiasm, I installed myself in my study to write the first pages of this, my latest book. I had been collecting facts, data and information for a long time and I was particularly keen on the idea of writing this book; as I love food, I was sure that it was going to be a pleasure dealing with this subject. My enthusiasm had increased during the time I had spent collecting and preparing the material for this study, partly because I came across so many misconceptions and incongruities concerning food. Yet it was also heartening to realise how many thoughts I shared with colleagues and other writers on this subject.

By lunchtime I had collated all the material I required from my researches. Without knowing that this was the day I had in mind for starting my book, my wife had prepared my favourite meal. It was actually very plain and ordinary, but delicious: an old-fashioned, typically Dutch meal – a hotpot of mashed potatoes with diced carrots and onions, with lots of lovely gravy; ideal nourishment for a cold winter's day. I thoroughly enjoyed it but once the meal was finished, I realised that I had over-indulged! Reclining in an easy chair I began to ponder the risks we run by eating too much: although food definitely lays a vital role in our lives, yet we must not underestimate the danger of its becoming an obsession.

That afternoon I felt too lethargic to leave my comfortable chair and make the effort to move to my study to start writing. Moderation in all things, I was forced to conclude, is a wonderful aim and yet, when something is particularly tasty, it is all too easy to convince ourselves that there is no harm in a little excess – hence the well-known saying: The spirit is willing, but the flesh is weak. Yet we don't need to look far to recognise the signs and results of obesity. For instance, just consider the high incidence of heart disease in this country. And this is only one of many problems which can arise when the body stores excess food as fat without giving the digestive system a chance of performing its duty. If too much food is eaten it can never be digested or assimilated properly. On such occasions we must conclude that food has become too important in our lives, and our common sense has been overridden by our greed.

Now I have confided in you that I like food, I must stipulate that I like good food. In truth, there was nothing wrong with the food I ate that day, as it was a healthy meal. But I over-indulged and by doing so my body was bombarded with too much of a good thing: energy was required and used which should have been channelled in other directions. It was utilised to overcome my lethargy and I wasted time before I could feel comfortable and regain my feeling of well-being: the result was that I lost a good part of that afternoon and pottered about without much achievement. Not succumbing to the temptation of over-eating, however, can sometimes seem almost impossible these days. We only need to look around our well-stocked supermarkets, delicatessen shops, restaurants, work canteens, coffee shops and snack bars to realise that we are spoilt for choice when it comes to food. What is not immediately obvious, however, is that these represent danger. Once we get used to the wrong foods or incorrect eating patterns it takes great determination to break the habit of over-indulgence, which we are all guilty of at times.

I often see this problem in patients who claim to be unable to control their craving and over-eat on a regular basis. By doing so, they sometimes actually cause themselves discomfort, by unplanned weight gain or indigestion, but they also increase the possibility of contracting heart disease. The heart in overweight people is over-taxed and has to work harder in order to perform its allotted and essential tasks. If we have partaken of a good meal, and have eaten in moderation, the results will be a feeling of healthy energy. We will feel replenished and ready to continue our work, not as I felt that day, when I felt depleted of the energy I needed to get on with the work I had planned.

The lesson I learnt at the outset of this book was worthwhile and it happened at a time when I could share my experiences with you. It reminded me that this is a widely recognised and experienced weakness, and I can share my concern with you. We must recognise the requirements of a sensible diet. A favourite saying of mine is 'There is nothing common about common sense', and it is with common sense that we must approach the subject of food, an essential and pleasant part of everyday life. The word 'essential' readily calls up unpleasant images but eating a healthy meal can be just as enjoyable as eating a meal from which our health does not benefit.

Just before starting this book, I had an opportunity to look around Arnhem and Nijmegen, where I spent my youth during the Second World War. This brought back many memories, but I could not help but remember how thin the people were in those days, especially during the last twelve months of the war. In the Netherlands the winter of 1944–45 is always referred to as 'The Hunger-Winter', because there was such a shortage of food. Even so, the tenacity and the energy of these people were much greater than you find in people today. I walked round a large supermarket in the town where I lived 48 years ago, and it was then, more than any other time, that I remembered the hunger and the emaciation of the people in the late war years. But when I looked around the supermarket at the shoppers and the shop assistants, I knew that yet again the health of many of those I saw was endangered. However, this time it was self-imposed. During the war, especially during the later stages, I saw people die of starvation, while today they die of excess. They die not only because of too much, but because the food is too rich and therefore it lacks health-giving properties. It is indeed a changing world. Let us remember the fact that half the world's population suffers from starvation. This is the real reason why I suggest that together we look at the negative and positive aspects of food.

Without doubt, the body is a wonderful and unique machine, an expertly designed piece of equipment. There are endless possibilities and variations in the use and maintenance of this equipment. Inherent characteristics can be destroyed by either giving too little or too much fuel or power, or by providing a power supply from the wrong source, i.e. by eating the wrong foods. Fortunately, in our Western civilisation it is rarely the quantity of food that is at fault, but sadly our food often lacks quality. I never tire of emphasising that we need food that is 'alive'. Until recently relatively little was known about the subject of nutrition or nourishment, but we are learning as we go along. Life is a chemical process. It all depends on the kind of chemicals we put into that process. Any form of life is a constant renewal of cells or cell tissue, while degenerative diseases mean a relentless breakdown of this renewal process. In fact, our health and energy levels depend on whether we use body builders or body breakers. This is the secret of life. Do we enhance cell renewal or, in our ignorance, do we encourage the erosion of life? The prime factor necessary for a well-functioning chemical process is that of high quality food and our diets should contain a good balance. Particularly in the case of illness and disease, a balanced diet is of prime importance. From the medical viewpoint we can hardly go wrong if we believe in the truth of the simple saying: food must be medicine and our medicine must be food.

Food ought to be eaten while it is fresh and it is important that it can be easily digested and absorbed. Especially in the case of degenerative diseases, the process of absorption is of great importance. Food should be seen as the fuel from which the body derives its energy. To the body, food is what coal is to a fire. The heat which is released in the body when food is being assimilated is spoken of in terms of calories. There are many different opinions on the permitted number of calories advisable to maintain good health and weight. On average it is thought that a person needs 2,500–3,000 calories a day, but it depends totally on the metabolism of the individual. Therefore I prefer a balanced diet which is worked out on an individual basis, according to one's individual characteristics and circumstances. I have patients with an excellent digestive system, who perform strenuous physical work, and they require in excess of 4,000 calories a day. By the same token I have advised others to restrict their calorific intake to 500–800 calories per day. It all depends on the individual's lifestyle and his use and requirement of energy. For more detailed dietary information I have decided to deal with fats, carbohydrates and proteins in separate chapters in this book.

Healthy eating means that we look for what will be advantageous to our own health. It is imperative that this is decided on an individual basis. Let me give you a simple example. The Italian diet contains much pasta, while the average Dutch diet contains a great deal of carbohydrate in combination with fats. This knowledge gives us an immediate indication of the likely cause of the many cholesterol-related problems in these countries. The British are well known for their sweet tooth, the Germans eat a lot of meat and sausages, while the French drink a lot of wine and the Americans have a weakness for beefburgers. Sometimes I sit in amazement in restaurants or hotel dining-rooms watching the eating habits of other diners and I have come to understand how such a large number of people have actively encouraged their bodies to become diseased. Adults, by not adhering to a sensible diet, actually solicit health problems, and there is no way that they can shirk the responsibility and lay the blame at someone else's door.

Carbohydrates are necessary and so are proteins, because they help the body to function well. But the body also requires food that contains vitamins, minerals and trace elements, and we often see that organically grown foods appear to enhance the body's well-being. Healthy eating is the result of rational and sensible thinking and some basic and essential nutritional knowledge. In my lectures to medical students I sometimes build up a picture of my imaginary house which I call 'The House of Health'. This is topped by the mind, as out of necessity this must be, and often is, stronger than the body.

With great interest I read recently an excellent new book called *Save the Earth*, by Jonathan Porritt. Reading through this, I was again horrified how, through the ages, we have set about destroying Mother Earth. I could not help but compare *Save the Earth* to other books on a similar subject, like Rachel Carson's *Silent Spring*, and the excellent publication by Gunther Schwabe, *Dance with the Devil*. I then realised that many things have changed since the earlier two books were written, and events across the world are progressively eroding human health. One message came across very strongly, and this I noted as I was determined to mention it in this book. Jonathan Porritt confirmed my belief that the mind is stronger than the body and a healthy mind will make a body as strong. Like me, he looked at the survivors. Even in time of famine and hardship the person with a determined character and inner strength often comes through such experiences a much stronger person. Good examples of such people were the survivors of the concentration camps at the end of the Second World War. Those who had the will to live often did so against the most dreadful and tragic background of human suffering. As far back as the days of the Old Testament, it was claimed that a strong mind could often overcome the influences of an incorrect diet. I have seen patients who survived serious diseases such as cancer, because their minds were strong and determined and they were willing and able to adapt to a healthy diet.

Healthy eating is more important now than ever before. When the first people on earth received the message to be fruitful, to multiply and to replenish the earth, they were also told 'to subdue it and have dominion over the fish of the sea, over the fowl of the air, and over every living thing that moves upon the earth'. As a naturopath I believe the most important aspect of life to be nutrition, and nature has supplied us with an abundance of first-class foods: fruits, vegetables, nuts, seeds, grains, herbs, etc. I have told you how I visualise my 'House of Health', topped by the mind. I have drawn a picture of a triangular roof for the house and have named the three angular sides as follows: mental, physical, emotional. Concentrating on these three factors should give us a healthy balance. Also, the house rests upon some very important pillars, five in all: nutrition, digestion, elimination, circulation and relaxation – working together these factors will provide an excellent chemical balance.

Healthy eating – how is it possible to emphasise its importance to our younger generation when they look to adults to set them an example? The many excesses witnessed among young children arise because their elders have seen fit to forget the laws of nature. I call upon mothers and grandmothers especially, and implore them to give their little ones 'live' food: forget the candies, sweeties and chocolates, and have a happy and healthy child. I never tire of emphasising this subject as it is very close to my heart. Thanks to my research work on a special project, I have had some close involvement with prisoners and have seen some of the repercussions of an unbalanced diet at close quarters. Many a criminal career has been launched when, as a child, a whine, a cry or a tantrum has been seen to produce a sweetie, resulting in a brief energy boost. If a child can continue this process somehow or another during its formative years and in later life, the sudden upsurge in energy as a result of adrenaline, sugars, alcohol or drugs can result in a bout of mischief, vandalism, etc., which eventually all too often results in a criminal record. This pattern of behaviour may have occurred during a person's youth and he may have grown out of it during his teens or twenties. If this is not the case he may have all the makings of a hardened criminal. Extensive research work on the aspects of crime related to diet has taken place in the United States, and is still ongoing. Dietary changes in institutions for young offenders, or borstals, have been established and the results are quite amazing.

Nowadays our health is under attack from so many different angles, due to environmental, traumatic, degenerative, genetic, viral and allergic influences. The 'House of Health' is attacked in many ways and yet common sense should allow us to approach this subject from the correct angle. The body triggers an alarm signal when there is something out of sorts. If there is a headache, there is bound to be a cause for it. When there is wind or flatulence, this will most likely be due to indigestion, which is a sure sign that something is wrong. Such deductions do not require a great deal of intelligence or medical knowledge. In the case of digestive problems the cause usually is found in the food that passes through the mouth, into the stomach, and through the duodenum. Our food must contain such ingredients as amino acids, glucose and essential fatty acids, which will make sure of good absorption and which, in the intestines, will separate into residual waste or influence the circulation. Blood, liver, heart, and in fact all internal organs, are dependent on healthy and wholesome food. It is an enormously complex chemical process which is involved here and a process which we should respect and learn to discipline. If we put our minds to it, we ourselves will be the first to realise how much better we feel on a change of diet and an added bonus can be the extra weight loss.

I have worked with people from all walks of life and among many famous people from the medical field, from the sports world and from the entertainment sector. Whenever I have felt that there might be something amiss with an individual's chemical process I have looked for possible problems in the cell renewal process, which would be a sure sign that his or her dietary management was defective. I have advised many people on the use of wholesome food, which must contain the essential nutrients, such as amino acids, glucose, essential fatty acids, enzymes, vitamins, minerals and oxygen. Once I am able to trace the missing factor(s), it is child's play to advise on solving the primary problem. It is simply a matter of introducing food containing the nutrients that are found wanting. With an improved diet the body will be encouraged to dispose more effectively of its waste material, the blood will be clearer, elimination will be improved, and the kidneys and lungs will work to our advantage. Our skin reflects what goes into our bodies and it also shows outwardly how healthy we are.

Sometimes I hear complaints that good food or health foods are so expensive. Let me assure you that they will always compare favourably with the cost of meat, which actually is a poor source of nutrition. Let me stress that in particular the older and the younger generation have a great need of wholesome food, in order to overcome tiredness, depression, poor complexion, digestive and absorption problems. Healthy eating also means regular meal times and proper mastication of our food. Saliva is the best digestive aid there is, but sometimes little or no time is allowed for our meals and food is hurriedly forced down with no proper chewing taking place.

The principles of correct food combining are very important and, even though I have stated this in some of my earlier books, I cannot resist the opportunity to re-emphasise that I have often seen digestive problems which were caused by eating carbohydrates together with proteins. There should be a break in between so that the body can easily digest these different nutrients. To eat a healthy diet is not really too difficult. Mostly it is a matter of mere common sense and the rewards will be more than worth our while. Overall life begins as a desire. To create a new lifestyle is an excellent desire to take better care. Nutrition is a subject that is vital to all of us: we are what we eat, and we are what we drink. The changes in nutritional value over the years have been dramatic, and many of us have lost the way.

When lecturing I hear questions such as, 'Why do you people all contradict each other?' It is then pointed out to me that there are so many dietary books which all lay claim to different methods to benefit one's health. Different speakers with excellent knowledge and qualifications in the field of nutrition are listened to and yet their advice always differs. I am fully aware of the confusing information, but a major yardstick must be that healthy food is food that is kept as natural as possible. We are being brainwashed by advertising in the press and the media, extolling the virtues of more and more cooked meals or half-cooked meals, which are supposed to be the answer to every housewife's prayers. Remember though: for food to be at its best it must be as natural as possible. When people are prepared to change their dietary habits and when they have followed my advice on specific dietary changes, they are delighted at the improvement in their condition. Take the example of my advice to arthritic patients who drink a few cups of coffee every day. When they follow my instructions and indeed stop drinking coffee, even if this is done for a trial period only, they come back and admit their disbelief that such a relatively minor change can have such far-reaching effects. I know that variety is the spice of life, but look at the riches of the nutritional kingdom: fruits, vegetables, plants, herbs, seeds, nuts and pulses. One soon realises that a healthy diet need not necessarily be a monotonous diet. The choice is ours.

Let us ask ourselves the correct questions: How many times a day do we eat fruit and vegetables? How many meals do we eat each day? How many snacks do we have in between meals? What is our daily salt and sugar intake? How regularly do we eat fish as opposed to eating a meat dish? How often do we eat fresh fruit? What is our liquid intake on an average day? When we answer these questions honestly, we will soon come to the conclusion that our dietary management leaves much to be desired. If we then remember that our bodies are alive we must surely begin to wonder why we insist on feeding our bodies with dead food. We want to be alive and healthy and therefore our choice of food must reflect that desire.

I have a good friend who is now the glorious age of 104, and I have known her for the last 26 or 27 years. In that time she has not changed very much and some valuable lessons may be learned from her dietary habits. She maintains that the relation of different nutrients establishes electromagnetic energies. If foods have the same energies, they will neutralise or destroy those energies, thus creating dead substances or substances without action. We must picture the body as a piece of equipment with electromagnetic properties. The acid/alkaline balance of the system must be judged on two levels: the fluids which control the ability of the digestive function and the cells which control the electromagnetic energies that regulate the digestion as well as the distribution of the nutrients to the cells. It is important that our food contains all the required minerals, including the rare trace elements, because it is the latter that form the ecto-enzymes, which act as co-enzymes and enzyme activators. These are not present in processed or over-cooked foods, nor in poorly combined foods. The minerals, including the rare trace elements, are the nutrients that create the electro-magnetic energies in food, and these combined factors control the acid/alkaline balance in the system. With this knowledge we must appreciate how important it is that we learn more about the chemistry of the body.

When lecturing I often point out that the body is like an energy field, with positive and negative poles. In blending acid and alkaline foods or drinks, we positively or negatively influence that field of energy. Energetic food, i.e. food that has life in it, will indeed affect health positively. My friend of many years, Dr Hazel Parcells, puts it as follows: 'These are the laws of nutrition with which the kitchen chemist must be thoroughly informed.' Many physical disorders and ailments have their roots in a wrong body chemistry and nowadays these problems are too frequently ignored. The symptoms we doctors sometimes see in our patients are often indicative of influences on the metabolism resulting from defective nutrition. If we consider how important the biochemical processes are in the living body and the effects of diet on a vast metabolic factory, we will realise that healthy eating will always positively affect any problems within the body, and will endeavour to get rid of toxic residues from food metabolism. A recurring migraine may well be an indicator that the liver is struggling to perform its task. The liver is the regulator of our health – one of the finest laboratories imaginable which every 24 hours manages to filter 1,200 pints of blood, day in and day out. If the liver cannot cope with the numerous waste chemicals contained in the blood, it will send out an alarm signal. A crisis point may be reached by a gradual build-up of insecticides we have eaten unwittingly with our food. The liver may send out an alarm in the case of an allergic reaction, possibly to pork or to chocolate, for example. We see the same thing happening with arthritis or eczema, and many other allergic reactions. Most of these conditions require an improved and healthy diet in order to change or reduce the level of toxic residue which will negatively affect the tremendous chemical process involved.

It is my experience that what is good for one person is not necessarily beneficial to another, and therefore I like to talk with my patients first and question them in order to decide which foods would benefit that particular person and, also of great importance, that person's individual lifestyle. Many people fall into the trap of eating foods they are fond of, which are rarely the most beneficial foods for them. A slight modification in the diet may result in a great change in a person's overall health and sometimes it is merely a matter of minor adjustment which can result in a significant change for the better.

In my studies and research I have paid special attention to groups of people who live in extremely remote areas where little contact has been established with the outside world. In those situations I have discovered a much lower incidence of disease and illness than is reported in western civilisation as a whole. In my opinion one of the major reasons for this is that these people live much closer to nature than we do and their food is wholesome and natural. The non-availability of processed foods is a benefit; they do not suffer because of the lack of these. I was impressed with the quality of the soil in which they cultivated their food and in the ways they worked their soil after harvest time in preparation for the next crop. At times we may regard such people as uncivilised, but with regard to their instinctive respect for food and their unspoilt lifestyle, we would learn a valuable lesson. To my way of thinking there is no doubt that here lies the secret of their longevity and their immunity to disease and illness.

Eating a wholefood diet means eating food as near to the condition in which it has been grown as possible, with little removed and even less added. Again, let's use our common sense: we cannot possibly eat the skin of a banana, as it serves to protect the soft inner fruit, but we can eat the skin of a potato, an apple, a tomato or a peach. If you cut a slice off a raw potato, for example, and hold it to the light, you can observe the mineral ring just under the skin and this shows how impossible it is to peel a raw potato without sacrificing some of these minerals. This then is the reason why I always advocate cooking potatoes in their skin. However, this is not a hard and fast rule, because in the case of carrots the situation is completely different. The mineral stores in carrots are captured more within the central cylinder and therefore it is desirable to scrub carrots well with a stiff brush or to peel the outer layer of the skin. This also applies when making carrot juice. Enzymes in raw food are important and that is why raw foods should feature in our daily diet – by having a salad every day we can ensure, as a result, that we absorb as many digestive enzymes as possible. It is also important to bring variety into our diet and to eat foods when they are in season so that they can be consumed in a natural state, instead of dehydrating, freezing or preserving them for use at a later time.

Don't always have the same things for breakfast, or for lunch. Do try and bring some variety to your diet, but for maximum benefit make sure that any changes or adjustments suit your way of life. Follow Adele Davis's advice that one should eat the heaviest and largest meal of the day in the morning, and that this should be the best meal of the day. In my clinic I see countless patients with digestive problems which concern me greatly. In most cases they have already been advised on dietary matters and yet they have chosen to ignore the advice and refuse to change their ways, or claim that they are unable to do so. In such cases the diagnosis of defective absorption need not come as a surprise. Alarms are triggered to alert us that something is out of sorts, e.g. excessive flatulence, bloatedness or swelling occurs – ideal conditions for the *Candida albicans* yeast parasite to become active. Often, however, such symptoms appear simply because foods have been wrongly combined, or too little attention has been paid to a good balance in the acid/alkaline system. If the digestion is good there will be little risk of distress. If the body lacks sufficient digestive enzymes, body language will tell us and we must learn to interpret the signs correctly and pay heed to the warnings. I have dealt with this aspect of health in my book *Body Energy* and it is nowhere near as difficult to understand as one might expect. Primarily it is a matter of common sense.

Another thing to aim for in your diet is to have at least 50 per cent of your food intake each day in a raw state. I know that this will not always be easy, but nevertheless it can be done. Just think of the opportunity at breakfast time! When fresh foods are in season have a bowl of mixed fruit, possibly mixed with muesli and pure honey. How about some beansprouts with wheatgerm, sprinkled with some nuts over the top for lunch? When you get into the way of things, you will find that it is not difficult to find suitable dishes of raw food. Think of the many varieties and combinations for salad and salad accompaniments. Maybe initially, a bit of imagination may be called for, but if you feel that extra help is required, there is a multitude of nutritional and cookery books to consult.

Healthy eating is balanced eating. The Chinese believe in the 'yin and yang' of food. They believe that before all creation there was chaos and that chaos was the result of undifferentiated energies in the universe. 'Yin and yang' – negative and positive – are natural forces in the world upon which all life is dependent. According to the Chinese one of the most important areas for a correct yin and yang balance is in the daily diet. For the Chinese the main dietary rule is to aim for a balance of five types of food: cold and cool (both of which are 'yin' or negative), warm and hot (both of which are 'yang' or positive), and, lastly, neutral foodstuffs. The modern Western dietary concept of nutrition is also based on five points. We have devised a system which accounts for five different groups: carbohydrates, proteins, fats, vitamins and minerals. In both schools of thought the correct proportions are important.

An interesting article was featured in the *Daily Mail* on Thursday, 25 April 1991. It was entitled 'Keeping healthy living in mind' and read as follows:

> 'If you want a youthful mind when you're 70, take a look at your lifestyle now,' say researchers.
>
> An investigation has shown that the mental ability of a middle-aged person in poor health gets worse quickly, while healthier over-55s experience only a slow decline.
>
> Professor Patrick Rabbitt, head of research, said: 'By

eating properly, not smoking at all, not drinking too much, taking exercise and by doing all those other dull things we are supposed to do – but few of us do – you are not just buying extra time, you are purchasing quality of life for your last 20 or so years.'

Fit older people can retain the mental skills of someone 35 years younger, he claimed, and there should now be a rethink on fixed retirement ages.

Psychologists at Manchester University's Age and Cognitive Performance Centre studied nearly 8,000 men and women between the ages of 50 and 96 – some for up to ten years – using lifestyle questionnaires and intelligence and memory tests.

Bear this in mind and decide to start enjoying a healthy diet which will provide us with a better chance of an enjoyable and worthwhile old age. Very few people will disagree when I claim that eating is an important and thoroughly enjoyable part of life. All foods provide some nutrients, but nutritional value will generally serve us better. In this book I intend to provide you with the information required for you to realise which nutrients should feature in a varied diet so that you can take charge of your own dietary requirements. If there is a good balance in our food intake, there should not be any weight problems. It is not an exaggerated claim to say that carrying surplus weight is quite rightly public enemy number one for our health. With a little imagination we can enjoy a healthy and richly varied diet without over-stuffing ourselves and sapping our energy. With a balanced diet, we will be able to enjoy our work, and have energy to spare for relaxing pastimes. Above all, remember the motto 'Prevention is better than cure'. Remember that with better dietary management it is possible to prevent illnesses and diseases. Life is a constant renewal of cells, and degenerative disease is the breakdown of life. Take the advice of Chuan Tzu, the Chinese philosopher:

The perfect negative principle is majestically passive.
The perfect positive is powerfully active . . .
The interaction of the two results in that harmony by
which all things are produced.

2

Fruit and Vegetables

IT WOULD TAKE something quite extraordinary to give me greater pleasure than a stroll through a well-stocked and maintained vegetable garden. It is a delight to see the range of different colours such gardens possess, to inhale and savour the smell of fresh and maturing vegetables, and ultimately to marvel at the natural treasure which has forced its way through the soil and is now available for our use and enjoyment. I get the same sense of elation and gratitude for nature's wonderful bounty when I wander through an orchard when the fruit is ripening and smell the heady aroma that makes one feel part of nature. From creation onwards, nature has endowed mankind with an abundance of foodstuffs containing all the vitamins, minerals and trace elements and much more which we require.

One of the most common questions fired at me when I have been lecturing is: 'Are fruit and vegetables really as good as is claimed?' We have a slight dilemma in answering this because the truth is that food's nutritional value is greatly dependent upon the quality of the soil in which it has been cultivated. This then opens the door to the next question: 'Are organically grown fruit and vegetables better?' Here I have no reservations and can readily answer in the affirmative.

One of our clinics is situated close to a nearby horticultural college and we have a good relationship with the college staff. We have worked out tables comparing the nutritional value of fruits and vegetables grown with the aid of fertilisers, herbicides, pesticides, etc. on the one hand with that of the produce cultivated in our organic nursery at the clinic on the other. It is quite fascinating to see how much higher the vitamin, mineral and trace element contents of the organically grown produce were when compared to those of the commercially grown fruits and vegetables. Selenium, calcium, iron, chromium, etc. were all much more in evidence in the organically grown fruits and vegetables, and this of course has important implications for our health. Such findings are often considered to be controversial and lack evidence. But there can be no doubt about the higher nutritional value of organically grown produce. This conclusion, added to the fact that fruit and vegetables grown in natural and organic fertilisers such as manure or compost derived from garden waste have a richer taste and smell, allows me to endorse wholeheartedly my belief in the benefits of organic gardening. Foods grown in soil fed with inorganic fertilisers such as sulphates, ammonia, potash and phosphates are of lower nutritional value.

We have also carried out a test with roses. A rose can give a beautiful scent. Yet roses bought from the florist often lack that heady scent which is present when they are grown in soil nourished with non-artificial fertilisers.

It is certainly true that in tests with patients I often find miasmas, usually the result of minute quantities of pesticides and artificial fertilisers which have not been cleared from the body; these are quite capable of adversely affecting their health. My conclusion is not based on an instinctive prejudice, but has been borne out by tests. From a medical viewpoint I am happy to stand by my statement that I endorse the greater benefits of organically grown vegetables and fruits as compared to those produced as a result of following commercial practices.

The Soil Association has very strict rules and this is something for which we should be grateful, because those rules are essential for the future. It is not always possible to prove the benefits of organic farming in scientific tests. But more than 30 years of experience has taught me that my claims are not idle ones. The fruits and vegetables grown in a good organic base contain immune properties and these characteristics are deposited and transferred to the human body. If we feed the human body well and try to avoid artificial ingredients in our nourishment, the chemical process that takes place inside us will serve us well. Artificial or foreign material may well be considered as an immune depressor and could affect the natural balance. Always be aware that a plant's produce is only as healthy as the soil from which it is derived. Sick soil will very likely produce sick plants. A further piece of general advice is that if at all possible fruits and vegetables ought to be eaten as raw as possible. There are edible plants found growing in the wild that can be very useful; some require to be cooked, while others do not. However, be very careful if you do not know what you are dealing with, because some species may be unfit for human consumption – certain kinds of fungi, for example are extremely poisonous.

One of the advantages of eating raw food is that it must be chewed very well. The action of chewing requires saliva, which is the best possible digestive aid. I often point out to my patients that deficient digestion and assimilation may be remedied by raw vegetable juices. I have lost count of the many stomach ulcers and acid problems I have helped to clear, for instance, with the simple advice of taking raw potato juice. So many patients have reported back in amazement, never having believed it was possible to find a cure for their ulcer or for their recurrent problems with psoriasis in as simple a treatment as drinking the juice of a raw potato (which neutralises acidity). With a diet of raw fruit and vegetables, or their juices, many deficiencies have been cleared. Most vegetables are rich in calcium and their characteristic is maintained in the juices derived from the vegetables. However, one must be careful not to allow the digestive system to become lazy. The chewing of raw vegetables is good for one's teeth and the chewing process is required in order that fibres and cells are able to release their nutrients. A well-balanced diet ought to include both raw and cooked foods, although in special circumstances it may be necessary to put the accent on raw foods, as when certain degenerative diseases are present.

At this point I want to stipulate one of the golden rules of food combining, a subject close to my heart. Always try to eat your fruits and vegetables at separate meals. Experience has proved that most people fare better on a diet which separates these two natural products. Alfred Vogel puts it nicely in one of his books when he says that 'our taste buds would hardly find a mixture of radishes and strawberries acceptable'. This is a warning for us to be careful. I will come back to my favourite topic of food combining in more detail in a later chapter.

Why do fruits and vegetables appear at the top of my list of dietary requirements? Apart from the fact that these foods are 'alive' there are two other good reasons: their fibre content and their nutritional value. Although some are more nutritious than others, all vegetables and fruits are an abundant source of vitamins, minerals and trace elements, and these gifts of nature are essential for good health. Individual fruits or vegetables may have special characteristics which are not common to others. For example, a grape diet encourages the body to cleanse and rid itself of toxins. Don't overlook the fact either that many fruits and vegetables have specific medicinal properties. Nowadays, although they are more specialised and cultivated, they can still fulfil a medicinal role. Wild vegetables are often of great use in this respect and in my book *Traditional Home and Herbal Remedies* I have written in detail about specific fruits and vegetables from the point of view of their nutritional value as well as their medicinal properties. We often see that people who live in out-of-the-way places, away from civilisation, are much more resilient to epidemics and illness, and often their main source of nutrition is wild vegetables. Living in a supposedly civilised culture, we could learn some valuable lessons from them concerning our dietary arrangements. It is not so much the quantities of fruit and vegetables we eat, but their quality that is of overriding importance here. I repeat that our food needs to be 'alive'; we are not dead creatures and we need 'live' food. The chemist Marcel Vogel, a well-known researcher in this field, stated in one of his lectures:

> Man can and does communicate with plant life. Plants are living objects and are sensitively rooted in space. They may be blind, deaf and dumb in the human sense, but there is no doubt that they have extremely sensitive instruments for measuring man's emotions. They radiate energy forces that are beneficial to man. They feed into their own force field which in turn feeds energy back to the planet.

It is fascinating to follow the growth of a plant, to study its development from germination to seedling and then follow its progress through various stages until it eventually blossoms, in readiness to bear fruit. If we take care of our fruits and vegetables, by properly working the soil and using natural manure, we will follow the laws of nature. This brings to mind the wonderful saying by Sir Arthur Eddington: 'When an electron vibrates, the Universe shakes.'

Yet another frequent question is: 'Can we eat what we want?' This is never an easy question to fob off with a partial answer. I try to explain that a good diet does not require any knowledge of mathematics. On the whole it is a matter of common sense. Common sense will tell us that if we eat a fruit pudding full of additives and colourings, the fruit in that particular pudding is doing us no good at all. When people, for whatever reason, lack the presence of the friendly bowel bacteria, a natural yoghurt may solve the problem. Unfortunately, in Britain especially, many people look at natural yoghurt as food for pigs, yet it is the most natural way of re-inviting some of these friendly, and essential, bacteria back into the bowels. They seem to have an aversion to natural yoghurt, but eventually will agree to buy one with added fruit. That would not present a great problem, if only a lot of other things had not been added in order to preserve the fruit in the yoghurt and keep it looking palatable. Often colourings are used in this process to produce what is considered by the manufacturers to be a more marketable product, and so a basically beneficial product is changed into something which has lost all its original nutritional value. A natural alternative would be to mash a soft, ripe banana through the natural yoghurt, perhaps adding honey to sweeten it. The end product would be most palatable without losing any of its beneficial characteristics. This is what I mean by common sense.

Life is a constant renewal of cells and to maintain life it is essential to regulate the intake of food, water and air, which in turn becomes body tissue. Under normal circumstances the bodily functions attend to the disposal of waste material. In this process the digestive system plays a major role, with the help of many other organs which in turn do their job in the overall metabolic process of digesting and assimilating the consumed food. All these organs together form a system that allows food and drink to be absorbed by the blood but in this whole intricate system it is often quite easy to pinpoint the source of digestive problems and thus concentrate on their removal.

In the first instance, every individual has a choice of what is allowed to enter the mouth and pass through the body. When the selected food has been chewed well, it is swallowed before it enters the digestive system for further processing. So far we have been in charge of this process, but from here on we have to leave the work to nature. The first actions are completely under our own control and we may think that we do not carry any responsibility for the remainder of the process. This is an incorrect assumption. We can actively encourage or even discourage the involuntary part of the process by taking an interest in what we eat and drink, and deciding on a sensible intake at any given time. In the case of problems, illness or disease, nature may require a little help, a subject I will return to later in this book with more specific examples.

The choice of food can be decided with the help of our intuition. Just as animals choose and instinctively know what they should not eat or drink, it seems that man once had this gift as well, but with the oncoming of civilisation we have moved further and further from nature's way and now our instinctive choice is decided according to our taste and appetite, rather than what might serve us best.

An interesting project was run at an American university with the participation of a large group of students. For several weeks these students were allowed a very extensive choice of foods. When they started the study their choice seemed to be very largely from the meat sector, but gradually a change of direction became noticeable towards a lighter diet containing more vegetables and fruits in preference to the meat dishes which required more effort from the digestive system. When quizzed as to whether this had been a conscious swing towards the more easily digestible foods, they claimed that they felt more energetic, and were generally feeling better, therefore they felt it wiser to concentrate on the foods that seemed to agree better with them. I wonder what would have happened if the choice had been towards more sugary products, such as cakes, cola and other products which were as readily available to them as the more natural foods. We know that sugar products can be very addictive and, although the natural sugar in food will produce energy and increase one's strength, sugar should not feature largely in anyone's dietary schedule. Diet should suit the individual and his circumstances and match his expected energy output. This must be taken into account when deciding on the 'best' diet for the individual. The most valuable piece of advice here must be to keep our diet as natural as possible. And with this statement we have turned full circle and are back to the beginning when I recommended that we rely on our intuition as to which food is good and which is bad for us.

'Is it better to steam vegetables rather than to boil them?' is yet another frequent, somewhat more practical question. Personally, I prefer my vegetables while they are still crisp. I do not enjoy vegetables when they have been overcooked and where possible I would advocate that vegetables are eaten raw. Second best to eating vegetables raw is probably steaming them. In the first place, steaming uses much less water. It upsets me to see vegetable cooked correctly, and then the water in which they have been cooked allowed to disappear down the drain of the sink. This water contains all the vitamins, minerals and trace elements which have been lost during the cooking and although this fluid would make an excellent stock to be used as a base for soup or gravy, mostly this is allowed to disappear down the drain. If you prefer to have your vegetables cooked until soft, please do not dispose of the cooking liquid, because the best characteristics of the vegetables have been transferred to that fluid during the cooking process. With steaming much less water is used and therefore less of the goodness has been allowed to escape from the vegetables. Pressure cooking is also recommended for the simple reason that the vegetables are cooked more quickly, and therefore they lose little of their nutritional value.

We now progress from the cooking of vegetables to the wisdom of cooking fruit. There are certain fruits that definitely require cooking, such as rhubarb, prunes, cooking apples and dried fruits. The golden rule here is not to overcook them. Dried fruits have a very low vitamin C content and by cooking them we are likely to lose even the little there was in the first place. The same goes for canned or tinned fruits. Too much of the goodness of the fruits is lost in the preservation process. Frozen fruits are certainly better than tinned or canned fruits. Heat treatment for fruits and vegetables destroys a tremendous amount of the quality. We need only look at the fruit in jams and jellies to see that little or no nutritional value is left after the preservation process has taken place. During the lengthy cooking process of the fruits with the added sugar most of the food value is lost.

Many plant cells have a tough cellulose wall and certain fruits require some cooking in order to get through the cellulose wall. In such cases a few minutes of boiling is often all that is necessary. A little while ago I was asked for my opinion on a book put together by *Reader's Digest* called *Eat Better and Live Better*. It was a pleasure indeed to be allowed to praise and recommend this book during a radio programme because much of what I read in it was in line with my own principles on dietary management. One of its main themes was that for most vegetables and fruit a little boiling or steaming only is necessary. We should not allow our food to be reduced to pulp before we are prepared to eat it. As a naturopath I was unable to agree with every assumption made in the book, but the widely varying menus which can be put together from fruits, vegetables, nuts, seeds, salads, etc. and the attractive dishes shown in that book are wonderful. Another interesting cookery book and one certainly worth mentioning in this context is *Cranks' Cookery Book* which, as the name implies, puts the emphasis on natural foods. In short, I would suggest that we have a good look at what can be done with the wealth of ingredients nature so readily supplies; the variety is infinitely bigger than one thinks. The more we experiment, the more ways of combining and preparing we will discover.

To close this chapter I would like to give you some basic advice on a cooking method for vegetables which ensures the minimum loss of nutrients from the fresh produce. The text for this is copied from one of the leaflets of our clinic which is given to patients who require dietary advice as part of their treatment.

The best way to cook vegetables is to sauté them in a round bottom Chinese wok. In this way the nutrients leached from the vegetables are retained in the vegetable juices. If vegetables are boiled, the cooking water should be retained as stock or thickened with arrowroot or cornflour, flavoured with mixed herbs and served on the vegetables as a clear sauce. If sea vegetables are sautéed with the land vegetables then the essential trace elements from the sea are brought into the diet in a very simple and natural way.

Vegetables are never as fresh as they could be unless grown in the back garden. To overcome this it is possible to grow fresh, nutritious vegetables in the kitchen all year round. Beans and seeds are easy to sprout, and as sprouts, because of their high nitrogen content, they are among the most nutritious vegetables available.

3

Pulses and Beans

PULSES AND BEANS are seeds of the legume family. These plants have the enormous advantage of nitrogen-fixing bacteria in the nodules of their roots and are capable of manufacturing large quantities of quality proteins. A pulse protein combined with protein from whole grains will give the perfect balance of amino acids for human requirements. Today, thankfully, they are quite rightly considered first-class proteins and not second-class, as was claimed until recently. These proteins will help the building of a healthy body and they are certainly of better value than proteins derived from animal sources. Without hesitation I advise my patients to invest in soya beans rather than in meat. When correctly prepared, soya beans can taste very good indeed and serve the body admirably. But it is possible to overdo things. Pulses ought not to be eaten with daily regularity or in too great a quantity. They are very filling and flatulence may result from pulses remaining in the intestines awaiting digestion and absorption. Furthermore, their preparation requires some special care and attention. The general rule for pulses is to soak them overnight before cooking. If this is done the soya bean, for instance, is one of the richest and most concentrated sources of protein and is nowadays widely available in the form of the popular Tofu – a truly versatile product that can be adapted to suit all imaginable purposes.

The legume family offers a tremendous choice of beans and pulses. They are tasty, versatile, look appetising and can be used on their own, added to soups, eaten hot or cold, and combined with many other nutritional ingredients. They are natural products with tremendous nutritional value, and represent a source of inspiration for the imaginative cook. For a while they seemed to have been pushed to the back of the shelf, but recently they have come into their own again. In the days of our mothers and grandmothers they were understandably popular as, due to transport limitations, the supply of fresh vegetables was more restricted. Fortunately, in a well-balanced modern diet they have again been accorded an important position. They are rich in fibre and also contain good quality carbohydrates and proteins, required for a healthy and strong body.

To prepare pulses, soak overnight. Take care not to overcook them, as they will turn to mush. Cover them with ample water, bring them to the boil and simmer them for about 20 to 25 minutes. Never add salt when cooking beans because this toughens the skins. By the time they are supposed to be ready, test them by pricking with a fork.

I can remember after the war, when we often ate pulses and beans, our great delight at having a square meal – my mother cooked them with onions and herbs and the end-product was delicious. If they are cooked properly, less flatulence or wind will be experienced, symptoms for which they are unfortunately notorious. Possibly this is one of the main reasons why beans temporarily appeared to become less popular.

Personally, I like all kinds of beans, but I am particularly keen on sprouted beans. There are many ways of preparing these attractively and they can look so appetising. Beans can be mixed with herbs, olive, almond or walnut oil, and they can be made into the most delicious soups or chillies. Lentils, of which there are so many kinds, have an equally good nutritional value and have the same health-giving properties as beans and pulses.

One good meal of pulses or beans can provide us with sufficient protein for a day. The soya bean is especially high in protein and, when it is crushed, a useful soya milk is obtained which in the Far East has been a staple food for centuries. The use of soya products is essential for vegetarians as, quite apart from their versatility, they are also a rich source of vitamins, minerals and trace elements. Tofu is a delicious substitute for meat, poultry, cheese, etc., and soya bean sauce is an excellent seasoning. With this information it will be clear why it is so necessary to use these excellent foods regularly in one's dietary schedule.

A large sector of the legume family is reserved for sprouting beans, grains, etc. Again their versatility is enormous, as is their nutritional value, which is second to none and promotes a good digestive process. Mung beans and alfalfa sprouts are the best known of the many in this group, but all can be used for more than one purpose. In order to understand the value of sprouting beans, a little about the digestive process must be explained. The stomach has six different sets of glands embedded in the mucous membrane wall. Here the enzyme hydrochloric acid begins the digestion of all proteins, whether these are derived from vegetable or animal sources. Pepsin, another enzyme, is also important in this digestive process, being a necessary acid medium to assimilate protein – a process in which gastric acid is undoubtedly a most strategic factor. As soon as a mouthful of concentrated protein is chewed, such as eggs, meat, fish, nuts or cheese, the stomach begins to go into action, prompted first by sight and taste, and followed by the secretion of HCl (hydrochloric acid) and pepsin.

The digestive process which occurs with sprouting beans, however, is quite different. These are an easily digested source of food. Although nutritionally satisfying, they do not leave the consumer with the terribly full feeling that may result from animal derived protein. They are a source of first-class protein and digestion can begin as soon as the food reaches the stomach. This process may continue for as long as two or two and a half hours, since protein requires relatively slow digestion. This partially digested protein is then passed through the small intestine and, aided by special enzymes, hydrolysis into amino acids is completed. It becomes obvious how well the body is equipped if nature is allowed to take its course and there is no interference. For instance, when a baked potato is consumed and properly chewed, only a low concentration of HCl is secreted. Between the stomach and the action of the intestine, 75 to 80 per cent of a starch meal is digested in the duodenum. The more mixtures in a single meal, the more complex are the demands of the body for complete digestion.

Large lumps of poorly chewed food may remain in the stomach and in the small intestine for longer and may even be impelled back for further digestion. Liquid, drunk while food is in the stomach, simply passes around the solid mass into the small intestine. Unless liquids are heavy or thick, such as milk, milkshakes or soups, they will normally leave the stomach within a few seconds of when they were ingested. Fruits, however, leave the stomach within a few minutes of the time when eaten and should be fully digested within one to two hours. Vegetables are processed only a little more slowly. Sprouts, on the other hand, are quickly digested and, in contrast to starchy foods and fats, which slow the digestion most, they are a tremendous source of vitamins, minerals and trace elements.

The stomach lining is protected against its own secretion of the protein digestor HCl and other enzymes by the flow of mucus across the surface of the lining, even though it has been estimated that for every gramme of protein digested and absorbed, an equal amount of protein is derived from digestive enzymes themselves and the mucus from the lining of the digestive tract. In order to reduce excessive mucus, which was often referred to as gastric catarrh, sprouted beans are excellent.

Sprouting can be done in several different ways, using many different kinds of seeds and beans, and therefore, as these also represent such a recognised nutrient in the Western diet nowadays, I want to spend a little longer dealing with them. Reproduced below is text from the BioSnacky brochure, produced by A. Vogel, containing useful and enlightening information, especially on some of the lesser known sprouting seeds and beans. This information will prove the versatility of sprouting seeds.

- *Alfalfa* sprouts have a slightly bitter, mildly nutty flavour. They contain among other things, vitamins A, B2, C, D and niacin as well as numerous minerals such as iron, magnesium, all eight essential amino acids, protein, chlorophyll and fibres.

- *Broccoli* sprouts have a delicate, aromatic flavour. They contain large amounts of calcium, chromium, iron, fluoride, iodine, potassium, copper, magnesium, manganese, sodium and phosphorus, as well as flavonoids, iso-flavonoids, glucosinolates, carotene, folic acid, vitamins B1, B2, B6, C, E, K, polyphenols and mustard oils.

- *Detox Mix* sprouts have a delicate, distinctive taste. They contain, among other things, vitamins A, B1, B2, B6, B12, C, E, calcium, iron, potassium, manganese, magnesium, sodium, niacin, phosphorus and zinc. Red Clover additionally contains so-called phytoestrogens (isoflavones).

- *Fitness Mix* sprouts have a subtle, mildly piquant flavour. They contain, among other things, vitamins A, B1, B2, B3, B6, B12, C and plenty of E. They also contain iodine, potassium, plenty of calcium, magnesium, manganese, sodium, niacin, pantothenic acid, phosphorus, sulphur and zinc.

- *Gourmet Mix* sprouts have a classic, delicate-tasting flavour. They contain, among other things, vitamins A, B1, B3, B6, B12, plenty of C and E, iron, potassium, calcium, magnesium, manganese, sodium, niacin, pantothenic acid, phosphorus, sulphur and zinc.

- *Little Radish* sprouts have a strong and spicy flavour. They contain, among other things, vitamins A, B1, B2, C, iron, potassium, calcium, magnesium, niacin, sodium and phosphorus.

- *Mild Aromatic Mix* sprouts have a light and delicate flavour. They contain, among other things, vitamins A, B1, B2, B3, B6, B12, C, E, iron, potassium, calcium, magnesium, manganese, sodium, niacin, phosphorus and zinc.

- *Mung Bean* sprouts have a mild and nutty flavour. They contain, among other things, vitamins A, B1, B2, B3, B12, C and plenty of iron, potassium, calcium, magnesium and phosphorus.

- *Red Clover* sprouts have a delicate, distinctive taste. They contain, among other things, vitamins C and E as well as essential oils, minerals and phytoestrogens (isoflavones), which are classed as secondary vegetable matter. Red Clover is particularly rich in isoflavonoids, which have a great affinity with female oestrogens.

- *Strong Aromatic Mix* sprouts have a strong, full-bodied flavour. They contain, among other things, the B vitamins, iron, calcium and high levels of protein.

Once you discover how economical and easy it is to grow sprouts, you will want to have some on the go all the time. Once germinated most kinds of sprouted seeds or beans can be stored in polythene bags in the fridge for up to a week – just long enough to get a new batch ready for eating. Most people grow sprouts in glass jars covered with nylon mesh held in place with an elastic band around the neck. Recently, an even simpler method has been discovered which allows you to grow many more sprouts and avoids the jar method problem of seeds rotting due to insufficient drainage. For this you will need:

- Seeds (e.g. mung beans).
- Shallow seed trays with drainage holes like those used in the greenhouse for bringing on seedlings for the garden. You can buy different sizes depending on how many sprouts you want to grow.
- A jar or bowl to soak seeds in overnight.
- A plant atomiser – available from nurseries, gardening or hardware shops.
- A sieve.
- Nylon mesh, also available from gardening shops.

The method of preparation is as follows:

1. Place two handfuls of seeds or beans in the bottom of a jar or bowl and cover with plenty of water. Leave to soak overnight.
2. Pour the seeds into a sieve and rinse well with water. Be sure to remove any dead or broken seeds or pieces of debris.
3. Line a seedling tray with nylon mesh (which helps the seeds to drain better) and pour in the soaked seeds.
4. Place in a warm, dark spot for fast growth.
5. Spray the seeds twice a day with fresh water in an atomiser and stir them gently with the hand in order to aerate them.
6. After about three days place the seeds in sunlight for several hours to develop the chlorophyll (green) in them.
7. Then rinse in a sieve, drain well and put in a polythene bag in the fridge to use in salads, to sauté on their own or mixed with other vegetables.

Seeds and grains are latent powerhouses of nutritional goodness and life energy. Add water to germinate them, let them grow for a few days in your kitchen and you will harvest delicious, inexpensive fresh foods of quite phenomenal health-enhancing value. The vitamin content of seeds increases dramatically when they germinate. The vitamin C content in soya beans, for example, multiplies five times within three days of germination – a mere tablespoon of soya bean sprouts contains half the recommended daily adult requirement of this vitamin. The vitamin B2 in oat grain rises by 1,300 per cent almost as soon as the seed sprouts and by the time the tiny leaves have formed, it has risen by an incredible 2,000 per cent. Sprouted seeds and grains also appear to have anti-cancer properties which is why they form an important part of the gentler method of treating the disease.

When you sprout a seed, enzymes, which have been dormant, spring into action, breaking down stored starch into simple natural sugars, splitting long chain proteins into amino acids and converting saturated fats into free fatty acids. What this means is that the process of sprouting turns these seeds into foods which are very easily assimilated by the body when they are eaten. Sprouts are, in effect, pre-digested and as such have many times the nutritional efficiency of seeds from which they have grown. They also provide more nutrients ounce for ounce then any natural food known.

Another attractive thing about sprouts is their price. The basic seeds and grains are cheap and readily available in supermarkets and healthfood stores – chickpeas, brown lentils, mung beans, wheat grains, etc. Since you sprout them yourself with nothing but clean water, they represent an easily accessible source of organically grown fresh vegetables, even for city dwellers. In an age when most vegetables and fruits are grown on artificially fertilised soils and treated with hormones, fungicides, insecticides, preservatives and all manner of other chemicals, the home-grown-in-a-jar (or tray) sprout emerges as a pristine blessing: fresh, unpolluted and ready to eat immediately by popping them into salads or sandwiches. As such they can be a wonderful health boon to any family concerned about the rising cost of food and the falling nutritional value in the average diet. Indeed, they must be the cheapest form of natural food around. Different sprouts mixed together will support life, all on their own. One researcher has calculated that by eating sprouts alone we could live on less than £0.20 per person per day. While I would certainly never suggest that anybody live on sprouts alone, I certainly do believe they are an ideal addition to the diet of every family – particularly if the housekeeping budget is small.

By the way, nearly all children love them since they can help grow them themselves. Also, because they grow so quickly – the average sprout is ready for the table in about three days – children's patience is not stretched for too long and their interest will be maintained.

Previously ignored, pulses and beans are a nutritional miracle. The vital natural forces hidden in pulses and beans will keep the body alert and alive in a truly natural way, and will aid our health by restoring and maintaining our immune system.

4

Nuts and Seeds

WITHOUT A DOUBT one can safely refer to nuts and seeds as rich sources of vegetable fat and protein. Excellent in small amounts, they deserve a place in everyone's diet. Everyone likes to nibble a few nuts, but have you ever thought of trying them in a salad, in baking, desserts, cottage cheese or with Quark? With a little imagination you will be able to find many more uses for them. Unrefined oils, such as olive oil, sunflower oil, soya oil, and the oil from nuts such as walnuts, pine kernels and even apricot kernels, contain a very high content of unsaturated fatty acid and research has shown how vital this is in our diet. Excellent supplies of unsaturated fatty acids are available even in the smallest of seeds, like the insignificant sesame seed, and their health-giving benefits are thus becoming increasingly recognised. In underdeveloped countries, where I have spent much time on research projects, it is amazing to see how extensively seeds are used. Sesame seeds, one of the smaller varieties, were seen as having magic properties as far back as 2350 BC, according to old scriptures. The Babylonians were known to make sesame wine, which was drunk for its pleasant taste, while at the same time it was recognised for its medicinal value. Indeed, sesame seeds always seem to have featured largely in the Middle East diet, both for their very pleasant taste and their health-giving properties. Way back in history, when the Greek and Roman soldiers went into battle, sesame seeds were part of their staple diet.

When sesame seeds are correctly combined with other nutrients they provide a balanced protein intake and for those who prefer meatless protein, sesame seeds offer a welcome alternative. They are rich in minerals, such as iron, potassium and calcium and are power-packed for rebuilding and maintaining health. The highly unsaturated acid of the sesame seed is easily assimilated in our cells and tissues and forms a very nutritious food substance. Not only are sesame seeds tasty, they are also a very good remedy for combating constipation, eczema and other bodily problems. Alfred Vogel prescribes the use of these little seeds for patients who suffer from liver and gallbladder problems.

As with all seeds, despite their size, sesame seeds must be chewed well. It is possible, when using an electric food processor or liquidiser, to make a lovely creamy mixture by blending sesame seeds with figs, apples, oranges, rosehips, honey or sunflower seeds.

It is comforting to know, in short, that even one of the least significant types of seed such as the small sesame seed, contains such vital power. That which contains life will always give life in return.

In the chapter on fats and oils, I mention the general lack of essential fatty acids in the average diet. Some of the small seeds which are readily available, e.g. blackcurrant, borage, evening primrose and sunflower, contain ingredients that are required for the creation and assimilation of the essential fatty acids which are vital to the body.

The plant that produces linseeds, *Linum usitatissium*, is one of the oldest cultivated plants in existence and is known to grow throughout the world. This small seed is extremely effective as a laxative and is invaluable as a natural stimulator of regular bowel movements.

Flax seeds have similar characteristics and, although they contain cyanogenic glycoside, there is no need to be concerned about poisoning since the Linamarasa splits to a slight degree due to the pH of the stomach. It even forms a protective layer over the mucous membrane, indirectly alleviating painful and inflammatory processes by its soothing and inflammation-blocking effects.

Mustard seeds are the smallest of seeds, yet are a useful digestive aid. They stimulate the flow of gastric juices. People who suffer from lumbago or rheumatic pains should take a hot bath to which some mustard seeds have been added; this they will find extremely relaxing. Female patients have experienced relief from vaginal problems after a warm bath with mustard seeds.

Coriander seed, which is so rich in vitamins and minerals, is also a marvellous appetiser and a very good remedy for the stomach. In olden days it was also used for rheumatism, painful joints and caries (decay of bones or teeth).

Pumpkin seeds have the most wonderful properties for men who have problems with the prostate gland. Many of my patients have been saved from surgery on this gland by following the simple advice of chewing a handful of pumpkin seeds every day. These seeds are light and nourishing, have a very pleasant taste and are a good source of the mineral zinc. Isn't this a much better way of overcoming a health problem than having to go into hospital for surgery?

The prime source of plant protein is nuts. It is very likely that nuts contain even more protein than milk, but of course they are much better for us. Besides protein, nuts also contain vitamins, minerals, salts, sugars, starches and oils. Moreover, the fat of nuts should never be confused with animal fats.

Nuts are easily digested unless they are combined with the wrong kinds of food. Animal products and processed foods are mostly incompatible with them. There is a tremendous variety of nuts available throughout the year, such as almonds, cashews,

Brazils, walnuts, coconuts, peanuts, hazelnuts, chestnuts and pecans. Personally my advice would be not to roast them, but to keep them natural, i.e. unsalted. Because of the many preservatives required much of their vital force is lost in processing. For health reasons they should be consumed in as close to their natural state as possible. Unlike seeds, one ought not to consider nuts as a suitable snack to have between meals. Nuts are really quite filling. And it must be understood that nuts are a little more difficult to digest than seeds and should be chewed very thoroughly. This should not present a problem, because nature has endowed us with teeth to grind, and nuts can be a plentiful source of nutrients, if only we take care to chew them thoroughly. Digestion of nuts is slightly more difficult because they contain certain enzyme inhibitors.

Let me tell you a story of a young man who adopted an all-raw-food diet and somehow decided that walnuts were to play a major part in this diet. He became ill and was greatly troubled with indigestion. It wasn't until he accepted the advice to ignore nuts totally as part of his diet that he began to improve. Until then, he had not been prepared to believe that the nuts were to blame for his condition because he had read that they were good for him. More than anything this little tale is a lesson in moderation.

The great Scottish explorer Joseph Thomson travelled extensively in Africa and was fascinated to learn that many of the natives existed happily on a diet of cereals, vegetables and nuts. These people's staple diet was made up of maize, root vegetables, green coconuts, sesame seeds and nuts, especially monkey nuts or groundnuts. Many kinds of nut aroused their interest, and because they were mostly vegetarian their diet was supplemented with honey, mango, pineapple and other fruits. The combination of nuts and honey was rather interesting because, whereas nuts are rich in protein and fats, honey consists of various sugars, mineral salts, iodine, phosphates, iron, calcium, magnesium, with some essential trace elements.

Many of these natural foods are coming into their own again these days, and I can only say that I am delighted. Just think how rich in nutrients the milk of a coconut is. I have prescribed this for some very severe degenerative diseases, like muscular dystrophy, and when it is taken together with supplementary amino acids I have seen some greatly encouraging results. Yet we cannot claim to have explored nature to the full. Take a look at the walnut, a fairly popular nut and recognised for its versatility. A chopped walnut in a salad tastes really nice, but inside the walnut we find a browny golden film, thin and fragile as tissue paper. For many years I have successfully used this for the treatment of diabetes, and have prescribed it often in combination with some other remedies such as Molkosan, and a bilberry extract from Alfred Vogel's range. Diabetics would do well to avail themselves of at least one pound of walnuts per week, break the shells and boil some every day and drink a little cupful; this will stimulate the pancreas to produce natural insulin. Quite a few of my patients had reached the stage where they had to inject insulin on a regular basis, but since following this treatment advice, they have managed with a course of tablets or are totally without medication.

Sometimes during lectures and talks I am asked to define science. To me science is about discovering the secrets of nature and making these available to man. The secrets of nature are very often hard to uncover and may be found deep down in little insignificant seeds that may contain some vital power, or even in the filmy membrane of the walnut, where yet another answer to some rather serious medical problems may be found. The question remains whether it is possible, taking into account all the investigation and the enormous sums of money that have been spent on medical research, that natural remedial sources have been insufficiently investigated or whether they have been overlooked as being too obvious. Sometimes a plant, a flower, a nut or a seed contains a wonderful secret of nature and may call out to us to be discovered, but I am doubtful if many of us have even bothered to look in that direction. These remedial and health-giving sources are widely accepted as food products, and we eat them unaware that they can maintain, increase and protect health from the many attacks that undermine our well-being today.

5

Starch and Fibre

IT MUST BE twenty years or so ago that a lady came to my clinic in search of a cure for a most unpleasant bowel problem. She told me that she had had problems for quite some time. I suggested that she ensure that her diet contained more fibre which would, through natural means, encourage bowel movements. She asked if I was sure that that was all there was to it and I reassured her that I was confident of my diagnosis and the treatment advised. It may be that because her husband was a medical specialist I thought I could detect some scepticism – she seemed to consider my advice too simple to be effective. In essence, I suggested that she enrich the fibre content of her diet by adding bran. When she got up to leave the consulting room, I knew that she was not overly impressed and I asked her to give it the benefit of the doubt and try a change in diet, even if only for a few weeks. She left after promising that she would give it a try. The next day her husband phoned and more or less ridiculed my suggestions; he implied that if it was as simple as that, he would soon be out of a job. I asked him to encourage his wife to try, because whatever his beliefs, there could be no harm in it. It must have been several months later when she again turned up at the clinic – with a beaming smile across her face. She was extremely grateful for the sound advice I had given her, because her problems had been solved. She also told me that I would be pleased to hear that her husband now prescribed the same treatment for his patients with problems similar to hers. I know that to this day her husband still advises his patients along these lines and now he has developed a great interest in dietary management.

Out daily diet must contain starch and fibre. These nutrients are filling without providing too many calories. In our affluent and indulgent society it is important that we eat filling foods which have good nutritional content, yet are unlikely to cause an increase in weight. A further benefit is that starch and fibre foods are usually reasonably priced and, as they are closely allied to carbohydrates, we will look at certain aspects of them again in a later chapter.

Wholemeal bread is a good source of fibre. For example, think of the Vogel loaf. For years now, this has been sold all over the world and it is packed with nutrition. The ingredients combined in this healthy bread supply us with almost a whole meal in a few slices. It's tasty, it's filling, but most important of all, it's very nutritious. The muesli breakfast also has lots of good fibre, being a mixture of fruits, oats, wholegrains, rice flakes, barley flakes, almonds, chestnuts, apricots, millet and durian. Durian is a tropical fruit which is excellent for the digestion. A breakfast of muesli thus supplies us with first-class energy. Consider ripe bananas, maize, millet, noodles, pastas, plantains, potatoes, rice, sweet potatoes, etc., and the myth that starchy foods are fattening will be destroyed. More than anything, the secret is the way in which they are prepared. A portion of chips, for example, has three times as many calories as an average helping of boiled potatoes. A slice of Vogel bread has about 60–70 calories and with a scrape of butter (which can be fattening) it won't exceed a total of 100 calories and is full of natural goodness. Its natural, simple nutrients provide a tasty but, more importantly, a healthy meal and help to prevent constipation.

Fruit and vegetables are also rich in fibre, and along with oats and beans will reduce the cholesterol level. I visited a health exhibition a little while ago in the company of the well-known broadcaster Gloria Hunniford. We walked around and looked at various things of interest and then arrived at a stand where a cholesterol count was being taken from a little blood sample. Gloria, who has a stressful existence because of her work as a broadcaster and television presenter, keeps to a healthy diet. The test concluded that her cholesterol level was average. On the other hand, I am the person who preaches healthy living and it was my blood sample that showed an above average cholesterol level. Immediately I understood why this should be the case: I had been travelling extensively and much of my travelling had been done by aeroplane. The food served on planes and in hotels tends to be richer than the food I would eat at home and I was indeed somewhat alarmed by the way my cholesterol level had risen. As soon as possible I changed my diet and for breakfast I chose oat bran. Every day I ate some grapes, chewing the pips thoroughly. It wasn't long before my cholesterol had come down to the acceptable 5.2 level. This is further proof that food can be of great help when something is slightly out of sorts with our health.

The circulatory system is very dependent on a healthy food pattern and if we were to ignore a situation with an increased cholesterol level such as I have just described, even if this was only a temporary basis, we would be inviting trouble. The circulatory system of an average adult contains about ten pints of blood and each drop of it is made up of 250 million red cells. There are also 400,000 white cells and 15 million smaller platelets suspended in the yellowish fluid called plasma. The condition of our heart depends on our lifestyle and on the foods we eat, and under normal circumstances, if life is ticking over at a steady pace and we are fortunate enough not to be under any real stress, each drop of blood passes through the heart and lungs once every minute.

During stressful times, or possibly while travelling by plane for example, this may increase to as often as eight times a minute. In our world today there are many health irritants, and therefore the white cells are very important because they fight invading germs, while the red cells carry oxygen from the lungs to the body tissues. Platelets are equally important and their function also depends on the quality of the food we eat. Blood plasma carries not only the red and white cells, but also other chemical substances. Ultimately, to repeat the statement I made in a previous chapter, our bodies are comparable to a chemical machine. The kind of chemicals we feed into that machine will decide our health and energy.

Conditions and lifestyle in the twenty-first century have rendered us more vulnerable to unfriendly and alien invaders and our immune system has become suppressed. It is a relief to know that blood plasma contains antibodies which help in the defence against invaders. Another of their functions is to rush to the rescue when we bleed. Then they assemble en masse and allow the blood to coagulate. Another twentieth-century development is the appearance of many viruses, and more recently that of *Candida albicans*. It is imperative, then, that we see how important it is that we follow a well-balanced diet, in order to strengthen and protect ourselves.

Because there are many different kinds of fibre, it is important to eat as big a mixture as possible. It is also vital that we drink plenty of fluids with fibres. Lack of fluids can cause a blockage. Bran is one of the richest sources of fibre, although it doesn't provide many nutrients. For maximum benefit we must make sure that our intake of bran includes other ingredients. Starch and fibre can be obtained from many other different sources which are made up of different chemical compounds. One such source is the pectin in fruit. Although not widely known, pectin contains useful properties for rheumatic and arthritic sufferers, similar to the properties found in cellulose in cereals and vegetables.

The outer layers of cereals and grains are very rich in fibre and that is the reason why I am so against the use of refined white flour. These important outer layers are removed in the refining process. In fact, they are sold as a separate food product, but it would be much better if the grains had been kept in their original state. All wholemeal cereals are good sources of fibre. Most nuts and fruits, as well as some vegetables, pulses and beans which have a high fibre content, have a high water content. This often means that one needs to take more for the desired effect. Not all vegetables have a high fibre content and in these cases it would be better to take some supplementary bran.

Fibre requirements vary according to each individual – if one has a lazy bowel, for instance, the fibre intake would need to be greater. I am convinced that this variation in each individual's dietary requirements was the reason for the controversy which was caused by a cereal advertisement some time ago. The slogan was: 'Keep the muscle, lose the fat and keep the bowels in perfect order!' It is not possible to retain muscle tone just by taking some extra fibre. It is not as simple as that. There are other requirements to take into consideration. It is unrealistic to make too many claims for one particular nutrient and this can be extremely harmful in the case of certain foods. I have tried to explain that it is near enough impossible to predict exactly how certain foods will be tolerated by the individual.

In Europe the daily intake of fibre ranges from half an ounce to one ounce and with this knowledge one is bound to be intrigued to see that a Vogel loaf contains slightly more than one ounce of dietary fibre. This is quite remarkable when we know that an average white loaf contains only about one-third of an ounce of fibre. Of course, it is always better to use brown bread as opposed to white bread. Without doubt, wholemeal bread is very much better for one's health, not only because it contains more dietary fibre, but also because it has higher levels of vitamins E and B, and a variety of minerals. The nutritious value of bread also depends on which grains have been used in the loaf and in which ratio.

Nowadays we see more and more people with wheat allergies, and in these cases it is much better to eat a special granary loaf which has a greatly reduced wheat content. If there are very severe allergy problems, it is better still to choose bread that is completely wheat free, or a gluten-free loaf may be preferred. These particulars are important. Wheat allergies present an ever-growing problem in that an ever-increasing number of people seem to react unfavourably to wheat: I will come back to this subject in a later chapter. If you are affected by wheat allergy a choice must be made from the various remaining types of starches and fibres.

Brown rice is always a sensible choice and when cooked correctly it introduces essential ingredients into the diet. Wholewheat pasta provides us with a versatile option and with the simple addition of herbs and tomatoes can be made into a tasty, nourishing dish. Further suggestions for pasta preparation can be found in numerous cookery books and therefore I will not go into further detail here. I am sure that many of you have already decided upon your favourite pasta dishes.

Dried beans, especially kidney beans, are often overlooked. With the exception of kidney beans, it is best to cook them slowly in a stew or casserole, in which case there will only be a minimal loss of vitamins, minerals and trace elements. Recently it has been discovered that kidney beans contain a toxic factor called haemagglutinin, which can cause severe gastroenteritis. This toxic factor can be removed by boiling the beans very vigorously for ten minutes.

People who become obsessed with weight-reducing diets often make many mistakes, mainly because such a diet frequently lacks fibre. Yet on a fibre diet it is easy to lose weight and there is no need to go hungry. Some time ago, Weetabix, one of the leading British manufacturers of fibre-containing cereals, published a special weight-reducing fibre diet, designed by a leading nutritionist, Dr Michael Turner, together with a home economist, Anne Page-Wood. The diet was based on the nutritional principle of containing a high proportion of nutrients and dietary fibre, and a low proportion of fats and rapidly absorbed sugars. It is a well-balanced and healthy diet which is hopefully still widely used. All kinds of allowances are taken into account and I have no reservations about encouraging people to obtain this particular diet plan, particularly if they have bowel problems. I do not intend to repeat the whole dietary plan here, but will restrict myself to repeating some important points it makes.

- Each day's menu has been carefully calculated to provide the right balance of nutrients.
- Do not add sugar to drinks or food. A low-calorie sweetener (saccharine, aspartame or acesulfame K) may be used instead.
- Always sweeten cooked foods (e.g. stewed or baked fruit) after cooking. Do not use sorbitol, fructose or any product containing them.

Bread
All bread and rolls should be wholemeal.
Alternatively, one pitta bread can be used occasionally.

Vegetables
Fresh or frozen may be used.
a) Assorted – 4 oz broccoli, courgettes, Brussels sprouts, cabbage, green beans, spinach, cauliflower, leeks and celery
b) Peas or sweetcorn – 3 level teaspoons
c) Root – 4 oz onion, carrot, turnip and swede

Potatoes
These should be baked, boiled or mashed (any milk or spread you might use must be from the daily allowance).
Small portion = 5 oz or 1 scoop of mash
Medium portion = 7 oz

Salad

Low calorie salad dressing may be used if necessary.

a) Green salad – as much as you like of the following: lettuce, cucumber, green pepper, celery, cress, endive, chicory, spring onion

b) Mixed salad – a selection of any of the following in addition to the above: tomatoes, bean sprouts, mushrooms, radishes, carrots, red or yellow peppers

Fruit

This may be fresh, frozen, canned in natural juice, stewed or baked without added sugar. One serving of fruit may be of any of the following:

a) Half a grapefruit or a medium-sized apple, orange, banana, pear, peach, nectarine, wedge of melon or watermelon, kiwi fruit or teo stasumas of tangerines

b) 4 oz of plums, raspberries, strawberries, blackberries, blackcurrants, pineapple, cherries or apricots

Pasta/Rice

This should be brown if possible. One serving = 1 oz uncooked weight.

Drinks

Milk added to tea or coffee must come from the daily allowance. Lemon tea, black coffee and all low-calorie soft drinks may be consumed as desired.

The manufacturers of Weetabix have done an excellent job in preparing this well-balanced, easy-to-follow diet. My only reservation is that it is not suitable for vegetarians and I sincerely hope that they might consider compiling a similar diet which is applicable to vegetarians, in particular avoiding the use of pork (which is a very acidic meat) and any of its derivatives. The inclusion of pork is the reason I cannot recommend it in my clinic.

A healthy diet will soon prove its benefits to the consumer. I call upon everyone to make a fresh start right now. Do not procrastinate. A fresh start does not necessarily mean that drastic changes are called for, because a small change may make a big difference. The choice we make in what we eat can result in the start of a happier and healthier life. A sensible and varied diet is important, but is even better if combined with some extra exercise and more time set aside for relaxation. This combination ensures a better quality of life.

Good sources of fibre (or roughage, if you prefer) are mostly inexpensive and there is plenty of choice. Just think in terms of the following:

- Two chocolate digestive biscuits have a fat content of 10 grammes.
- A slice of wholemeal bread has a fibre content of 2 grammes.
- A beefburger has a fat content of 19 grammes.
- 4 oz of baked beans have a fibre content of 8 grammes.

Starches and fibre should always be chewed well. The action of chewing, because of the enzymes released in the saliva, encourages the digestion. Our teeth were meant for chewing, not only for smiling, although this is a good bonus. Increased mastication and therefore salivation will ensure proper digestion and, equally important, good absorption. One of the hidden benefits of wholefoods is that they are mostly chewy foods. In an article in the *Daily Mail* on 22 August 1991, a reporter by the name of Newby Hands wrote that the 1980s was the decade of good health in its great emphasis on books, supplements, etc. In the 1990s we saw a reversal and now nutrition is the watchword; the realisation is that long-term good health depends on a sensible, balanced diet. Nutrition holds the secret of our future. Today we read about pollution, stress, fertilisers, pesticides, and quite clearly these are identified as problems of the 1990s. The obvious consequence is that food or vitamin supplements may become increasingly necessary. On the other hand, the body has its own language and the cure is within. A wise old doctor once said: 'All curing is within the body itself.'

6

Fats and Oils

IT'S A FEW years now since I met Ude Erasmus, the writer of the book *Fats that Heal and Fats that Kill*. We had some interesting discussions about his work and his convictions and came to the conclusion that we were in total agreement on the problems and misconceptions about the place of fats and oils in the diet. We had some interesting discussions about his work and his convictions and came to the conclusion that we were in total agreement on the problems and misconceptions about the place of fats and oils in the diet. I can still remember that after the Second World War people insisted that it was essential for the diet to contain a good deal of fat. Of course, this was a gross mistake but all kinds of fats were consumed to enable emaciated people to regain some of the weight that had been lost during the war years when food had been so scarce. Before too long many health problems started to emerge. Nowadays the dangers are even greater in that in the past people performed more strenuous physical work, and the fats and oils in their diet served to give them muscular strength and energy; because of the circumstances, fats and oils were burnt up more quickly. Nowadays too often wrong fats are used and these are unfortunately stored somewhere in the body, endangering our future health.

Although the language may appear complex when we talk about triglycerides, cholesterol, saturated, unsaturated, mono-unsaturated and polyunsaturated fatty acid chains, the explanation for why we need much less of certain types of fats is easy to grasp. The message from the Royal College of Physicians, in this context, is clear: reduce your fat intake.

In my book *Heart and Blood Circulatory Problems* I have written in considerable detail about the role of cholesterol and I do not intend to repeat this here, since I would expect that by now we all know that cholesterol is a major contributory factor in cases of high blood pressure and heart disease.

Some points are worth repeating, though. The other day a female patient asked me for help and advice on how to get rid of her cholesterol. Smilingly I told her that if I did as she asked she would be dead. We all need a certain amount of cholesterol, and it is only when the level of cholesterol and triglycerides gets out of hand that we have a problem. During a radio interview recently I was joined by an eminent physician from the United States and we agreed that an ideal figure for cholesterol would be 5.2. Possibly this may be stretched to 5.5, but definitely no more than that. We must bear in mind that anything higher than 5.2 should be considered a warning that we are creeping up to an unacceptable level. People wonder if there is any reason why among the Yugoslavs and the Italians the incidence of heart disease is relatively low, certainly compared with our statistics. Think of the amounts of olive oil these nationals use in their diet and yet no damage seems to be inflicted on their health. The conclusion must be that olive oil does not have an undesirable effect on their cholesterol level. Now look at the situation in Great Britain. I quote an article from the *Daily Mail* published on Tuesday, 6 November 1990:

DINERS WITH FAT CHANCE
OF A RIPE OLD AGE

More than 180,000 people a year die from illnesses which could be prevented by healthy eating, a leading Government expert on nutrition said yesterday.

Britain is turning into a nation of fatties and people are still choosing the wrong food, said Dr Martin Wiseman, head of nutrition at the Department of Health.

Dr Wiseman was speaking at a conference held by the Consumers' Association as part of its healthy eating initiative, aimed at encouraging chefs in restaurants, schools and works canteens to include healthy options on their menus. Dr Wiseman said nearly half of all men and more than one in three women were now overweight. 'In 1980, we had 39 per cent of men overweight and 32 per cent of women overweight,' he said. 'Those figures have risen to 45 per cent and 36 per cent. This is a significant increase and these people run a substantial risk of developing illnesses.' England, Scotland, Wales and Northern Ireland were all in the top seven in a league table of death rates from coronary heart disease in 23 countries, he added.

'One hundred and eighty thousand people in the UK die each year from preventable heart attacks and strokes. There is a strong correlation between these diseases and the poor British diet. There is little evidence that the British diet is changing that much. Each British person still has a diet that maintains 40 per cent of saturated fat. These people have to be made aware that there are healthy and interesting alternatives.'

One of Britain's leading cardiologists, Sir John McMichael, challenges the claims that changing diet, reducing fat and cholesterol can change the incidence of heart disease. Vast sums of money, he claims, have been spent in the research of cholesterol reduction, whether it is by diet or by drugs, and it is time to admit that these efforts have not had the desired effects on the incidence of coronary heart disease. I am astonished. I need look no further than at the patients who attend our various clinics. They are all the proof I need to be convinced that when the diet is correct the cholesterol level drops.

I agree that besides diet other factors must be considered, but nevertheless diet is one of the main contributors towards high cholesterol levels and this must be taken very seriously. People must be made aware of what is beneficial to them and what is not; most people actually have little knowledge about nutrition or diets. Weight reducing diets, yes, because one rarely opens a magazine or a Sunday newspaper without reading about yet another diet which will make the weight drop off. However, on general dietary matters relating to nutritional value or basic knowledge about the role and the need for vitamins, there is much the general public should, but does not, know.

Occasionally I ask patients if they know anything about the carbon change of fatty acids, about essential fatty acids, or about polyunsaturates, and I admit that I find their general lack of knowledge quite disturbing. One lady told me that she knew for a fact that butter is fattening and that it is considered better to use margarine. I certainly feel rather nonplussed at times. I know that the margarine manufacturers spare no efforts to promote their claim that butter will cause the cholesterol level to increase. Their campaign has been so successful that this is now widely believed. But if we look at the composition of some brands of margarine, they are ten times worse than a scrape of butter, which contains digestive enzymes to facilitate proper digestion. Frequently I point out to patients that I would suggest they use small quantities of butter in preference to a poor quality margarine that has been subjected to a process which I cannot recommend. Butter is made up largely of fatty acids, called buteric acids, and it has only four carbon atoms. This means that it will dissolve easily in water on a low melting point of eight degrees Celsius. Hence a little butter is easily dissolved in the blood and is therefore burnt up and digested quite quickly.

In a normal diet, on average about 40 per cent of the digested calories are retained. It is important that the digestion and absorption of fats and oils is such that the correct nutritional breakdown is possible and easily achieved. This is the reason why saturated fats are harmful in the body, while polyunsaturates can be of help to the digestion. Polyunsaturates rarely contain less than 16 carbon molecules, while mono-unsaturates may contain as few as ten carbon atoms.

Eating foods that contain fats or oils is necessary for a proper metabolic function and they are also required components for our hormones and tissues. A measure of fat and oil in the diet is essential and the absorption of fats deserves as much consideration as the digestion.

In several of my books I have mentioned the importance of essential fatty acids, such as oils from the evening primrose seed, blackcurrant seed, borage seed and flax seed. Combined with fish oils, essential fatty acids are capable of performing a wonderful job and they are a prerequisite for good health. As far as degenerative diseases are concerned. I have researched multiple sclerosis in detail and I have seen some wonderful results as a result on the increased intake of essential fatty acids. I have also seen much degeneration and illness because of a deficiency of fats and oils. In the case of multiple sclerosis it intrigues me that there appears to be such a high incidence in the Shetland Islands, where fish is considered a staple part of the diet. Shetlanders have a similar culture to the inhabitants of the Faroe Islands, and I am puzzled as to why multiple sclerosis is virtually unheard of there. Both groups of people have a similar sort of lifestyle, yet on the Faroe Islands the diet contains more essential fatty acids and is more varied than that typical of the Shetland Islanders. The Shetland Islanders eat a one-sided and monotonous diet, and this may well be the answer to the puzzle.

On a similar note we discover that people who suffer from exhaustion or ME are advised to check their diet on the intake of protein, fats and carbohydrates. Often there can be a link if deficiencies in these nutrients are discovered and this could well be the underlying cause of the problem.

Over the years I have been consulted by many sports people, among them well-known footballers and golfers, and I have counselled them on dietary needs. Their way of life is physically very demanding and they are looking for optimum strength, stamina and fitness. The other day, in a book called *Fats, Nutrition and Health*, written by Dr Robert Esman, I read that in the 1920s an American scientist, Professor Meyerhoff, discovered that all biochemically active tissue is based upon a combination of sulphur-based amino acids and dietary essential fatty acids. It is, in fact, these dietary components that I have always recommended to my footballers, golfers, etc.

How much fat should one eat? In truth, we do not need very much, but the little we do need should be fat from the right source. Fatty foods are more compact than other foods because they contain less water. Fats provide more energy than carbohydrates or even sugar and my old friend and partner, Alfred Vogel, has stated that 30 grammes of fat per day is sufficient. If we think back to our biology or home economics lessons at school, we remember being taught that most foods contain fats or fatty acids. Remembering that, we must understand that we ingest much more fat than our body requires.

When contemplating a reduction in our intake of fat, one's first thoughts go to the obvious sources, such as butter, margarine, lard, etc., but believe me when I say that these constitute only part of the problem. Cream, chocolate, cheese, milk, and even cakes and biscuits, for example, all contain significant amounts of fat. The other day I read the label on a container of sheep's yoghurt and was amazed to see how many fats are contained in a small tub of this product. The same applies to other animal produce, particularly to pork and all its derivatives, such as sausages, bacon, ham and gammon. The fat content of pork or products derived from this source is unbelievably high. If one is not prepared to forsake such products, at least be prepared to take into account the best method of preparing them, i.e. by grilling. When bacon and sausages, for example, are grilled much of the fat is in fact lost. Sometimes, when I explain to patients preferential ways of preparing food in order to reduce their fat intake, they take fright and ask if it would not be better if they banished all fat from their diet. No, certainly not, because our diet needs a certain measure of fat, but let's try to eat smaller quantities of the correct fats. The golden rule is that any balanced diet ought to contain a certain amount of essential fatty acids.

In his interesting and educational book which I have mentioned, Ude Erasmus explained that unsaturated fats can be separated into three categories: Omega-9, Omega-6 and Omega-3. The omega number shows where the first double-bond on the fatty acid change occurs. The Omega-9 variety is one of the main fatty acids. This is found in many nuts and also in olives. In contrast with Omega-6, the former is very important for the metabolism. In some illnesses and diseases a combination of linoleic acids is recognised – these are found in nuts and seeds, especially linseed, safflower, sunflower and soya beans. Just as important is the gamma-linoleic acid (GLA) which is found in borage, blackcurrant and evening primrose seeds. Of course, other fatty acids are necessary, but it is important that these three omegas are available in the body, this being an essential requirement in order to achieve a good dietary balance.

Babies sometimes lack fatty acids and if this defiency were to continue for long periods, it might exhibit itself in eczema or general growth problems. Whilst adults have fat stores in the body, babies do not have this reserve.

One of the principal reasons why fats and oils should be included in the diet is that many contain vitamins, such as vitamins E and D, which are essential; therefore my response to whether or not we should include fats in the diet must be affirmative, with the stipulation that the quality and quantity is of overriding importance. Similarly, essential polyunsaturated and linoleic acids should be included. These act as body builders when they are of the correct quality, while they must be regarded as body breakers if the quality is poor or are derived from an incorrect source.

Let me give you a quick recap of the difference. The majority of fats used are from animal sources, i.e. meat, butter, cheese and cream, which contain few polyunsaturates, but are rich in saturated fatty acids. We need either very little or none at all of these saturated fatty acids, but it is beneficial for us to have polyunsaturated fats. Mono-unsaturated fats such as olive oil are not very commonly used, and yet they are very valuable in a balanced diet. The saturated fats are very hard, and the polyunsaturated and mono-unsaturated fats often look like liquid. Let there be no misunderstanding: all edible fats are a mixture of different fatty acids, in varying proportions.

Recent studies have shown a relationship between excessive use of fats and the increased occurrence of coronary heart disease. I frequently visit the United States for lecture tours and I have noticed that this subject always seems to cause great interest at my lectures. Actually it should not surprise me. When I look around me in the many hotels and restaurants which I have frequented there on my many travels, I can well understand the concern about cholesterol problems and coronary heart disease. Dietary imbalance in relation to fats and oils is still a relatively unknown subject to many people in the US. Sometimes I think that in Great Britain we don't fare very much better. The generally high intake of saturated fats here is very worrying. I have seen it mentioned that in Britain more than 45 per cent of the daily diet contains fats and oils, and if this were true, we certainly have a devastating statistic on our hands. Unless the fat intake is drastically reduced, problems will come sooner rather than later. There is much to be learned on this subject by the average person. For example, since hard margarine is a mixture of animal fats and vegetable and fish oils, one would be inclined to think that this must be better than butter. However, unless the margarine is of top quality, a hard margarine can be more harmful than a scrape of butter. We must learn about nutritional value and we should use the information that manufacturers are obliged by law to put on the levels of their products.

People are sufficiently aware to think of eggs, kidneys and liver as cholesterol-rich foods. But do not confuse the issue by believing that a reduction here would solve our problems. This is the first step only. To improve our health, saturated fats must be recognised for what they are. As a general rule we must discontinue the use of any hard fats, i.e. fats that remain hard even at room temperature. A further piece of information is that cooking oils or fats should never be reheated. After use they should be disposed of and not used again.

Without doubt, I can assure you that over the years I have seen the benefits of a vegetarian diet in old age. Let me just point out that my dear friend and colleague, Alfred Vogel, was 94 years old and still fit enough to ski. This was only a single example as an indication of his excellent general health. For the dedicated meat eater I would stress that he or she look for varieties of meat that are low in saturated fats or, better still, contemplate a move towards eating more fish, because fish in general is low in saturated fats and yet at the same time the body will be provided with the fatty acids that are needed.

The same rules apply to dairy products. Consider the difference between skimmed milk and milk straight from the cow. When grilling cheese, look at the difference between the quantity of fat that drips from Cheddar cheese and compare this to the fat which drips from Gouda or Edam cheese. The Dutch housewife will tell the cheese merchant, 'I want 40 plus', and then she thinks that she has a good fatty cheese. I can tell you that on the same scale Cheddar cheese comes in at least 80 per cent fat content; when we have a toasted cheese sandwich and much of the fat of Cheddar cheese has dripped away, it therefore seems foolish to congratulate ourselves that we have done quite well because this is less harmful than eating Cheddar or Cheshire cheese in its original state.

We must use our common sense about how we prepare food. Trim off any visible fat, remove skins from chicken or game and grill the fats out. When opening a tin of fish, such as sardines, tuna or salmon, do not mix the preserving oil through the fish but throw it out so that we can at least avoid these extra fats. Whenever possible food must be grilled. I know that in the Netherlands people like a fry-up and sometimes rich food is fried up the next day with the addition of even more fats – this indeed could induce carcinogenic conditions.

When preparing a salad dressing, remember that a very tasty dressing can be obtained using olive oil, or sunflower oil mixed with some Molkosan. Never forget that when we eat too much fat we increase the chance of health problems. When I study the diets of cancer patients it is often obvious that some of their problems have been of their own making. The body stores excess fat and in the case of overweight people, excess fats and oils can cause further unnecessary deterioration in their health. Energy is needed to perform our daily work and this is provided by eating the right foods; we need foods that supply us with energy instead of foods that deplete our energy – energy builders and not energy takers. But we should never eat more food than is needed for our energy requirement.

An informative little book has been written by Dr Elizabeth Evans. Because of the author's common sense, I would strongly advise my readers to read this book, which is called *Diet and Nutrition*. It contains some very useful tips on dietary management and should be helpful in finding a happy balance in your daily food and drink intake. Such a balance is especially important in a world in which our tastes have been greatly influenced by the large range of processed foods available. Walk around a supermarket or a food store and look at the exotic and enticing food products that are displayed. Think of the nutritional value of these. Do not be fobbed off by manufacturers' claims, but scrutinise the labels of what you buy ands what is available on the shelves. Free-range eggs are not only better for our health, but are also tastier. The nutritional value of fresh fish or fresh fowl is so much higher than that of processed fowl, or frozen or tinned fish. The Eskimo diet contains many fats and oils, but these are fully unsaturated and not harmful towards their health. Eskimos have a surprisingly low incidence of cancer and this could well be because they eat so much fresh fish.

In my book *Life Without Arthritis* I have drawn attention to the Maori diet. It is not their present state of health that is so impressive. I put the clock back some 40 or 50 years and studied their diet as it was then. They took fish from the sea, cooked them in the hot water of the geysers, and their general health as a result was outstanding. Their respect for natural food was exemplary. They were the best fighters, the best dancers and the healthiest people in the world, because of their lifestyle and the strong immunity towards diseases they developed. Basically, however, it was the way they prepared their food and kept their fats and oils in an unspoilt and natural state that was the decisive factor. Their diet replenished energy rather than depleted it. The contrast between their diet and ours could hardly be more striking. We do not seem to realise that the function of fat in the body is to provide us with muscular energy and the extra fat in our bodies is probably only for the purpose of padding and protection. Protein and carbohydrates are easily converted into fat, with, of course, the difference that linoleic acid is not produced. However, one does not need much of this. I repeat that in many countries, as is the case in Great Britain, an excess of fat is ingested, more often than not of the wrong kind. It is quite clear that both the Maoris and the Eskimos treated their raw fat in the way they dealt with their raw food. And because it was raw it was much less dangerous.

Vegetable fats are much better than animal fats, because in vegetables, fats are a natural substance. In tests it has been concluded that polyunsaturated vegetable fat and oils have no link to heart disease and coronaries. The minute quantities of vegetable oil contained in grape seeds on the other hand, have been a blessing to countless people all over the world. I advise people to eat a handful of grapes every day and by chewing the pips or seeds of the grapes, the vegetable oil in the seeds will be released and will set about depressing the cholesterol level. By doing so some of my patients whose cholesterol had been measured at between eight and nine have managed to reduce this to a level of around five.

However, let's not oversimplify the matter. Never think that the warning against saturated fat bears no relevance to unsaturated fat. It is never wise to eat or use too much of anything, no matter how healthy a specific ingredient may seem to be. I have seen people who have zealously adhered to dietary instructions and have concentrated on eating polyunsaturated fats only, thinking they were doing the correct thing. By doing so they have not succeeded in alleviating existing health problems, but worse still, they have inadvertently caused other problems, as a high intake of polyunsaturated fats can lead to an increased risk of degenerative disease. So be moderate in all dietary matters and a sensible and a balanced diet will be rewarded. Prevention is always better than cure and we can prevent much illness and disease by using common sense in order to get the optimum energy from the right fats and oils.

7

Fluids

THE OTHER DAY I read an advertisement for yet another brand of lemonade with the accent on its health-giving qualities. Out of interest I bought a can and it wasn't until I came home that I read the label. In amazement I read it again and was struck by the thought that all this 'health drink' was suitable for was cleaning my car windscreen. There are many beverages which are body breakers as opposed to body builders. The body needs plenty of fluids, but it needs good quality fluids. One of the best drinks is WATER. Even here it's sometimes difficult to get a good quality product as this life-giving fluid is so badly interfered with nowadays. However, the body needs fluid since without it we would not be able to survive for more than four days. It is particularly galling then that, in some areas today, it is said that we are drinking the nation's processed sewage and that we would do better to drink distilled water. Yet, once water has been distilled it has no life in it; it would be better to opt for bottled mineral water, which is pure, has life in it, and is a good body builder. Like normal water, it is also a perfect liquid for the blood.

The best sources of water are those which are available from pure supplies and certainly not those from dirty lead pipes. In my own house I have the problem that the water coming from the taps is often an unpleasant brown colour. Every time I phone the water authorities they go to great lengths to reassure me that the water has passed all the tests and there is no harm in drinking it. Sometimes the water loses its brown tinge and turns opaque milky white. It rarely seems to have the clear look which it is supposed to have. Yet pure water is an all-important factor in everyone's diet and consequently water filters are often necessary nowadays. It is necessary to ensure that the water we drink does not endanger our health and we should find out what sort of processes our water has been through before we drink it. In my book *Water – Healer or Poison?*, I have set out more detailed information regarding water filters and also my suggestions for keeping the water supply pure.

When you are thirsty, water is the best thirst quencher. It is good to dilute the natural enzymes in the stomach by drinking water. A glass of water should be drunk two hours after a starch meal, four hours after a protein meal, 30 minutes after a fruit meal, and 15 minutes before any meal. Always let the water from the tap run in the morning before using it, and whenever there is any doubt in your mind, phone the local water authorities to ensure that the supply is as pure as possible. It is always important to have access to a supply of good quality water, but never more so than when illness and disease has struck, and if in any doubt, please restrict yourself to bottled mineral water.

There are a few other things I would like to make clear, although in my book on water I have given plenty of specific advice. As a general rule, never fill the kettle from the hot water tap, because that water will have been heated the previous night and allowed to cool down before being reheated. The mineral content will have diminished and will diminish further still while the water is being boiled. Always empty the kettle after use and when boiling water is next required, refill the kettle with water from the cold tap. Water can be a healer and yet it can also act as poison.

Even with mineral waters you must be selective. Some contain high levels of sodium and other salts which are capable of causing harm. Still water is sometimes more beneficial than sparkling mineral water. You are what you eat, but you are also what you drink.

In those areas of Britain where fluoride has been added to the drinking water, please be extra cautious. Fluoride can be harmful, and there is strong evidence that it can be a body breaker. Good healthy teeth can only be attained by chewing food well and eating plenty of raw food, which will build up a natural fluoride protection. The role of fluoride in our water supply and the problems caused by it are discussed in the book *Fluoride* by Dr Hans Moolenburgh, and translated into many languages. Fluoride is not only a cumulative poison, but it strongly suppresses the immune system. In certain areas adverse affects have been reported, but the authorities cannot and will not believe that this could be due to the addition of fluoride to the drinking water. It is important that we are selective with respect to the water we drink. We need fluids, but they must be the right ones.

I have mentioned before that I once wrote to the Minister of Health asking why he did not put a laxative in the water, because half the British population appears to have constipation problems. Part of the problem is caused by the use of salt and medication taken by people who are ignorant of the dangers of taking the chemicals involved.

My great friend and co-lecturer, the late Dr William Ellis from the United States, was a man for whom I always had great respect. He left us with some sensible advice and allowed me to use some of his ideas. The following paragraphs reflect his thoughts and are worth bearing in mind:

> Fluid is essential throughout our bodies. Primarily, it is essential in the bloodstream to maintain the right consistency. It is very important in the bowel. If there is insufficient fluid in the bowel the result is constipation.

Kidneys require fluid to filter all the waste products efficiently for disposal.

To maintain body fluid levels, the amount one should drink is variable. For example, when the weather is very hot and we perspire through our pores, fluid loss increases, and it is necessary to drink 10–14 glasses of fluid daily. This can include fruit juice. It is important to remember that fruit juice is only fresh for about seven minutes after it is produced. This is because it has a hydrogen ion content, which is in the form of a gas. This evaporates and thereafter the vitamins, minerals and trace elements diminish and deteriorate. It is the same with vegetable juices. After seven minutes the juice has deteriorated so much that it is only valuable for its fluid content.

Beverages are also important. Most people drink too much coffee. Unfortunately, coffee is a strong diuretic and it acts on the kidneys, impairing the filtering function. Coffee causes the kidneys to eliminate potassium and the vitamin B complex. Decaffeinated coffee is even worse, as nickel is used in its production. We have found high levels of nickel in people who drink decaffeinated coffee. There are plenty of excellent healthy coffee substitutes.

The same rule applies to tea, as it is also a diuretic. It is far more beneficial to drink herbal or fruit teas. These are completely natural, full of flavour and extremely refreshing. Mint tea is very good for anyone with digestive problems as it contains pepsin. Pepsin acts as an activator on the cells that produce acid in the stomach. A shortage can cause or aggravate constipation.

I now follow on with some of Dr Ellis's thoughts regarding milk. In a subsequent chapter on protein I will spend some time on this subject, but I thought it best to keep Dr Ellis's ideas together.

Milk is probably the most common allergen, together with chocolate and cheese, which contains large amounts of phenylethylamine. Here you probably have the biggest single cause of migraine.

Human milk is acid, but the milk from cows and goats is alkaline. Human babies are born with an enzyme called rennin in the stomach. This enables then to digest their mothers' milk. Calves have an extra stomach called the milk stomach, but in order to digest their mothers' milk they must suck from the teat which produces the digestive enzymes.

When infants are weaned, the mothers' milk dries up, because there is no longer stimulation. For a cow to keep manufacturing milk, the pituitary needs to be stimulated, which in turn stimulates the mammary gland. The pituitary hormone is a growth hormone, which is obviously passed on into the milk, and then onto the consumer. In adults it is said that only 50 per cent produce a lactose enzyme in order to digest lactose sugar, which is the sugar found in milk. No wonder milk can be responsible for so many problems.

I would like to finish this section of the chapter with one of his favourite sayings. I have often heard him finish his lectures with it, and I have borrowed it from him before now: 'It's a case of mind over matter; no mind no matter.'

A positive mind will act positively. This is seen so often with another fluid which has become a big enemy – ALCOHOL. Alcohol is responsible for many problems and one has to be extremely careful with its intake. It is not a body builder, but without a doubt a body breaker. Alcohol is a fluid which is not nutritional or even helpful. It always affects the liver and will damage the brain enzymes as well. The expression 'Good health' when a strong drink is consumed is ironic. Alcohol undermines health, and unfortunately in our present-day affluent society often becomes compulsive. In some cases people are even in the habit of taking a liquid lunch, and are then unable to do their work in the afternoon. Frequently, people become dependent upon alcohol because of the stress and strain of modern life, depression, unhappiness, work resentment, marriage problems, etc., but alcohol only aggravates these problems. Alcoholism is becoming a universal problem and we certainly should be very cautious with the use of this fluid. Brain damage can be a result as alcohol affects the thalamus; it will also place pressure on the liver, which is already overburdened. One should not be ashamed of ordering a fruit juice or a soda and lime instead, if alcohol is becoming a real problem. There is no need to wait till one realises that a problem has arisen with alcohol before switching to soft drinks. Unfortunately, too often a soft drink is considered unmanly or unsociable. This, of course, is absolute nonsense.

There are many drinks which are said to be beneficial, but let me tell you that there is nothing better than a freshly extracted juice. Can you think of anything nicer than a fresh pineapple, mango, papaya or orange juice? These are real body builders, unlike the more popular beverage COFFEE.

The other day I met a man who refused to pay for treatment or remedies for his arthritis. I had told him some months ago that if he didn't want to pay anything, but wanted to get rid of his gnarled and knobbly fingers and wrists, he should stop drinking coffee. Coffee, you see, is acid forming and, as Dr Ellis often says, 'People put coffee into the wrong end'. Coffee is an excellent enema, but certainly not a good drink. Not only is it very addictive, it does much harm to the body and causes over-acidity. The sodium in our body works together with potassium, producing better fluid flow and maintaining the correct fluid balance in our cells. Because we consume excess sodium, often in the form of salt, even although we eat nearly as much potassium derived from fruit and vegetables, there is a tendency to accumulate sodium in our cells where we should have potassium. The result is that cells become swollen with water, because salt attracts water – and this can lead to heart attacks. A potassium-rich drink in the form of a substitute coffee is therefore very necessary and one of the finest to my knowledge is Bambu coffee. Bambu is rich in potassium since it contains chicory, figs, wheat, barley and acorns, and it makes a very pleasant drink. Created originally by Alfred Vogel, it has been enjoyed in Europe for over 40 years now and in a recent consumer test of favourite alternative beverages gained 80 per cent of the vote. It is worth adding that we must also be careful that decaffeinated or substitute coffees contain beneficial ingredients. Otherwise substitute coffee can be just as bad as normal coffee.

Contrary to popular belief, we also have a big problem with TEA. Tea-drinking has always been a wonderful social custom, but the tannin in tea is definitely not beneficial. There are of course teas that do not contain tannin. Moreover, there is a great choice of delicious and aromatic herbal teas, such as chamomile, peppermint and rosehip. The added bonus with these natural or herbal teas is that they can even be of medicinal help. I have used a combination of several herbs in a recipe which is greatly liked by many of my patients. Not only is it a refreshing and healthy recipe, it is also of tremendous use medicinally. It is made according to a recipe that is over 150 years old and has proven itself many times. It contains, in fact, 15 different kinds of the finest herbs, carefully selected, and is without additives, artificial colourings or harmful substances.

Directions for the Jan de Vries Tea

– Colds and Flu: One cup four times a day
– Rheumatism and Arthritis: One cup three times a day
– Skin Problems: A few cups per day
– Stomach Disorders: A few cups per day
– Tiredness, lethargy: Four to five cups per day
– Slimming: Several cups of this tea per day will help weight reduction by removing excess fluid

The regular use of this Herbal Health Tea can being relief to many ailments, aches and pains:

Red Clover:	Blood cleanser, alleviates bronchial coughs
Skullcap:	Benefits the nervous system, aches, pains, insomnia, rheumatism, female cramps, colds, fevers, exhaustion, heart
Chamomile:	Benefits stomach, colds, bronchitis, headaches, bladder troubles, rheumatic pains, nerves, hysteria
Passion Flower:	Anti-spasmodic, benefits neuralgic pains, nerves, convulsions, nervous headaches
Alfalfa.	Blood purifier, benefits wind pains, backache, sinus, dropsy, kidneys, arthritis, peptic ulcers
Lavender:	Prevents migraine headaches, baldness
Comfrey:	Benefits coughs, kidneys, bowels, stomach, rheumatism, blood in the urine, indigestion, eczema
Strawberry leaves	Blood purifier, benefits liver, gout, sore throat, arthritis
Dandelion:	Benefits liver, skin diseases, loss of appetite, kidneys, dropsy, fever, hepatitis, gout
Peppermint:	Benefits stomach, indigestion, convulsions, liver, diarrhoea
Hawthorn:	Benefits heart, insomnia, high blood pressure, stress, arthritis, rheumatism
Juniper berries:	Benefits kidney, bladder, prostate
Rosehips:	Prevents colds, flu, benefits bladder, spasms, kidneys, nervous headaches, palpitations
Golden Rod:	Astringent kidney cleanser
Salvia:	Benefits menopause problems, colds, sweating

Lots of people ask me what I drink myself – I love the Swiss Molkona drink, which is not only very good for the stomach and digestion, it also is very refreshing. As a child my mother gave us buttermilk to drink, which is also good in that it contains a lot of digestive enzymes, as Molkona does, but the latter is a better and healthier drink, and more refreshing.

There is a huge number of fluids available. If we take care and are selective, our reward will be energy, good health and happiness.

8

Proteins

THERE IS A great misunderstanding that all proteins are excellent body builders. I agree that some proteins are body builders, but there are also proteins that are body breakers. I am involved in several nutritional research projects and am often asked to explain the nutritional difference between proteins and carbohydrates. This done, I am often accused of showing a preference for carbohydrates. I only have to consider diets in some of the countries I have visited, where animal protein is in relatively rare supply, to see the relative advantages of carbohydrates. It is mostly the case that people who consume proportionately less animal protein work harder physically and have more strength and stamina than people who eat more. In Europe and the United States in particular, protein intake is far too high, particularly animal protein intake. I often review patients' diets in order to re-educate them and encourage them to balance their food intake. I grade fruits, vegetables, nuts, etc. as first-class protein sources, and usually patients experience a big improvement in their health when following my advice to increase their intake of these. As I mentioned before, I like to refer to such types of food as being 'live'; meat, milk and eggs, on the other hand, are sources of 'dead' protein. When I worked in the inlands of China I realised that the protein intake of the local people was no more than 40 or 50 grammes a day. Yet in China I was never consulted by patients with high blood pressure; there it is a most uncommon affliction. In countries where the people have a high protein intake it is much more common. In my book *Viruses, Allergies and the Immune System*, I point out that high protein intake causes mental stress. A high protein intake can also be the cause of digestion, absorption and constipation problems.

Alfred Vogel has a nice analogy with respect to protein and carbohydrates, when he compares the consumption of food to stoking a fire. He reckons that taking protein foods is like burning coal on a fire. When the coal has burnt, among the ashes we find clinker and stones in the grate. So it is, in a sense, with animal protein: we often see the evidence in the joints of arthritic patients. Carbohydrates, on the other hand, burn like wood. Wood burns up cleanly and leaves nothing but powdery dust. Carbohydrates are digested and leave the body without leaving deposits. In this context I must again reiterate that whatever is imported must be exported within 24 hours. If any remainder is left behind, problems will result.

There are a few foods that may be considered as major hazards of health and one of these is MEAT. From the point of view of food combining we know that meat is a difficult protein to digest. The dead protein we eat, from animals, birds, etc., is of little use to us. We are living beings and therefore we should eat 'live' food. Animal-based protein is absolutely dead.

We are not equipped to deal with large amounts of meat. The real meat eater, or carnivore, will thus develop a completely different type of intestinal bacteria to that of the non-meat eater. In the animal world it can be clearly seen that a meat eater, or carnivore, has been given long and sharp teeth for tearing flesh, while man has teeth that really belong to a herbivore or grain eater.

There is also a considerable difference between animal saliva and man's saliva. Man's saliva contains ptyalin, which helps the digestion, while an animal's saliva has ptylin. Furthermore, a meat eater has at least ten times more hydrochloric acid in the stomach than a non-meat eater. When man bombards his stomach with meat he poses a problem for his digestion. Certainly the hydrochloric acid required is greatly increased because animal fats and acids unbalance the acid/alkaline system. With this in mind, I strongly oppose the use of any kind of pork or pork produce. Pork is a particularly acidic meat.

A meat eater must always take more and better care than a non-meat eater. One would indeed be better without meat altogether, but if you are unwilling to give up meat completely, undoubtedly the safest meat is lamb. Fish would be better still, while beef should be eaten as an exception rather than as a rule. Personally I prefer pulses, grains and vegetables and would encourage you to decrease meat consumption and gradually introduce pulses. The crucial point is that your intake of animal protein should be reduced.

It appears that worldwide there is a general reduction in meat consumption. Yet in the *Scotland on Sunday* of 17 November 1991 I read that the beef industry has set aside the grand sum of £1.3 million for a promotional campaign called 'Meat to Live', aimed at increasing demand for their produce. In this particular article it was claimed that meat was essential for a healthy diet and could provide health benefits superior to those of balanced meat-free diets. I repeat that anything that lives needs to be kept alive with 'live' food. The article went on to make a reference to Henry VIII who, the reader was informed, celebrated a birthday party every day, with every imaginable kind of meat dish. Just what health benefits this particular example was meant to demonstrate I am at a loss to say. More than £8 million a year is spent on promoting meat nationwide, however, and for the last five years, despite this, there has been a considerable reduction in the £2 billion annual beef turnover.

According to a consumer poll on attitudes towards meat published in April 1991, 43 per cent of those polled claimed to have reduced their meat consumption and 10 per cent said they have now become vegetarian. This is a welcome trend. Fat and meat are both empty foods and do not contain the health properties claimed by the campaigners. The dripping roast on Sunday or the crispy bacon or ham sandwich may smell delicious, but in time will probably disappear, as dead food cannot nourish and sustain life.

In Scotland the incidence of bowel cancer is higher than anywhere else in the world. Is this surprising when we learn that the average meat intake is also highest in Scotland?

During a person's lifetime animal protein intake may reach such heights as seven to eight head of cattle, 36 sheep, 36 pigs, 750 poultry, and a few dozen rabbits and other game. By contrast, in an article in the *Scotland on Sunday* of 29 September 1991, it was mentioned that in the Middle Ages meat was only ever eaten in small quantities and even then on feast days only. I can say with confidence that meat will have to disappear from our diet, not just for the sake of our health; we should also take into account the suffering of animals in order that we can eat meat. Too much animal protein is wasted. A complete protein intake can easily be built up by food combining. Eating pulses and cereals, seeds, nuts, and some dairy products should be preferred. Sometimes meat eaters try to excuse themselves and say that they eat only fowl or game. It is not always the actual meat or fowl product which is harmful, but the hidden additions in them – many chemicals and by-products are now used at random by farmers. This results in a very suspect end-product. I have a patient who has worked in the meat market for nearly half a century. He told me about the changes he has seen and the difference between meat today and 30 years ago. Over the years he has become a very selective meat eater and tells me that he cannot enjoy meat unless he knows where it has come from. 'It's shocking what cattle breeders inject into their animals,' he told me; it is also shocking to learn how chickens are reared and prepared for the retail market.

According to an article in the *Daily Telegraph* of Friday, 19 April 1990, uncooked chickens and frozen birds very often contain salmonella bacteria. Out of six chickens examined five were found to be contaminated. Furthermore, 16 public health laboratories in various parts of the country co-operated in obtaining 146 frozen and 146 chilled chickens from a variety of sources, including supermarkets, butchers' shops and grocers. Seventy-nine of the frozen chickens (54 per cent) and 62 of the chilled birds (42 per cent) contained the salmonella virus – an average contamination level of 48 per cent. We ought to be aware of such dangers. Many kinds of tests and research are done on dead animals, but are they all safe and effective?

In a further article the *Daily Telegraph* claimed that a special diet for cattle, aimed at increasing their milk yield as effectively as giving them a hormone injection, has been developed at the Hannah Research Institute in Ayr. The Institute is exploring the discovery that protein fragments in the gut can increase nutrient intake as much as bovine somatotrophin, a hormone declared safe by the European Commission. Yet, in Britain, this hormone has caused concern over its long-term effects. Sometimes we must wonder what is going on. How can we trust scientists? Can we claim that what is produced and presented to the customer is safe for consumption?

On the subject of what is and is not good for us, I would like to say that I wholeheartedly agree with the contents of an article in the *Daily Telegraph* of Friday, 19 April 1991, by Virginia Matthews, which is worth quoting here:

DOCTORS 'FAIL TO PASS ON SENSIBLE EATING DATA'

Doctors are 'useless' at talking to their patients about diet and nutrition, the chairman of the Coronary Prevention Group said yesterday.

While the medical profession was adept at shaping

attitudes to health among professionals, it had proved to be 'clumsy' at educating people they treat, added Prof. Philip James. Speaking at the launch of a healthy eating campaign, targeted jointly at doctors and the general public, he said the future health of Britain was too important to be left to doctors. He took both the Government and the food industry to task for their apathy towards Britain's 'chronic' inaction over diet-related disease.

Although the Department of Health and the Ministry of Agriculture sent 'warm wishes' to the campaign, they have offered no tangible support, such as money.

The campaign – backed by the Consumers' Association, Coronary Prevention Group, Guild of Food Writers and the National Federation of Women's Institutes, with support from the Health Education authority – insists that eating healthily does not mean self-denial.

Recent World Health Organisation findings suggest that, despite relative affluence, Britons have an over-average risk of a number of diet-related diseases.

The campaign report finds that Britain has among the highest rates in the world of heart disease and breast cancer and suggests that these should be reduced radically with only limited changes in diet and lifestyle.

The backers of this report fear that the key WHO findings, disseminated with great interest among doctors, have failed to be 'pointedly and forcefully' put to the people who need to understand them – that is, the consumers.

Coronary heart disease kills one in four Britons resulting in an annual death toll of 180,000.

The campaign action plan includes:

– Better nutritional education in schools

– Compulsory and clear labels on food with
  nutritional detail
– A choice of healthy foods in restaurants and
  canteens
– Supermarkets and retailers to offer shoppers a
  wider range of healthy food.

This campaign deserves all possible help and encouragement and one can only hope that the organisers will be successful.

I agree that we need protein, but we should realise that we can easily live on 40–50 grammes of protein a day. Protein is, as suggested, available from meat, fish, eggs, dairy products, seeds, nuts and grains, and is essential in our diet in that, of the 22 known amino acids we require – amino acids being the units into which we break down protein – eight cannot be manufactured by the body and must be taken from food. Most grains, nuts, seeds and legumes need to be combined to make a complete protein. Forty to 50 grammes of protein may not seem a lot, but is the equivalent of 12 oz of yoghurt, or two to three eggs, which of course is far too much for one day. If the body takes in too much protein, it struggles to burn it up, especially if it is of animal origin. If the burning-up process is not efficient, it could result in the development of poisonous by-products. To prevent this, always make sure that most of the protein is eaten at breakfast time.

To promote the production of intestinal bacteria to aid digestion, it is very important to eat a portion of natural yoghurt daily so that the balance of friendly bacteria can be maintained. For a really healthy breakfast, mix yoghurt with a mashed banana and wheatgerm. For a change you may want to sprinkle it with sesame, sunflower of pumpkin seeds. Any of these combinations gives an excellent protein-based and tasty breakfast. Each one can also assist in maintaining a proper alkaline/acid balance.

Essential fatty acids such as linoleic and gammalinolenic acids are important for the skin and also help to control cholesterol levels. Proteins such as cheese and eggs can be very acid and therefore I rarely recommend these. Eggs may be high in vitamins, minerals, lecithin and cholesterol, but the lecithin is destroyed when eggs are cooked in fat or oil. Eggs boiled, baked, or fried in a non-stick frying pan without oil, would be a lot better.

Fish is an excellent protein because it is easily digested and broken down in the intestine where vitamin D is formed and it is also high in essential fatty acids and minerals such as iodine. Remember that good nutrition is the key factor in maintaining a healthy lifestyle and taking care of our health doesn't need to turn us into health fanatics: sometimes we need only rethink our values. Very many people have benefited by replacing meat with fish, and in doing so they have reduced their cholesterol level. If one is not prepared to be a committed vegetarian there is still no harm in occasionally replacing a meat-based meal with a vegetarian-orientated meal, which at least reduces fat while increasing fibre in the diet.

The latest surveys show that about one person in four takes vitamin, mineral and trace element supplements of some kind or another. These range from low to high potencies and there are numerous different combinations. Every now and then people worry about their diets and wonder if they are deficient in nutrients. In order to protect themselves from horrid diseases they take all these supplements, but conveniently forget that there is nothing better than a well-balanced diet. When I see patients with minor problems, these can be indications of deficiencies and I advise them to pay extra attention to their diets, supplementing them as recommended in the chapter on vitamins, minerals and trace elements. Prevention is better than cure and the long-term benefits of health supplements do help to protect us and should be considered a good investment. Unfortunately, because of the way our food is grown and treated nowadays, many deficiencies have to be rectified by such means. Think of the younger generation with their hankering for junk food, especially beefburgers. I was handed a leaflet produced and distributed by Animal Aid in London, entitled 'Burgers – What are you eating?'. Although it does not make entertaining reading, I have decided to include the text as it may make us reconsider a few established facts.

Ingredients of 100 per cent beefburger
30 grammes flaked or ground beef shin (including gristle, sinew and fat)
16 grammes beef mince (including heart, tongue and more fat)
10 grammes mechanically recovered meat (MRM) obtained by stripping the remains of the carcass and grinding the bits into a fine slurry
20 grammes water
2 grammes salt and spices
1 gramme monosodium glutamate and colouring
5 grammes polyphosphates and preservatives

'The meat industry relies upon pharmaceuticals to ensure that animals reach the slaughterhouse alive; kills them in conditions where hygiene standards resemble a poorly maintained public lavatory and then relies upon chemicals to make the finished product look and taste edible.'

Mark Gold, *Living Without Cruelty*

A recent survey showed that one in four burgers on sale in the EEC contains residues of banned growth-promoting hormones. Beef cattle are routinely dosed with low-level antibiotics and in recent years they have been fed slaughterhouse by-products. Waste from the carcasses of cattle, sheep, pigs and hens has been recycled into the feed, both of their own species and that of each other. Cattle and sheep are herbivores, they are not scavengers and have little defence against viral infection from food. The effect of this unnatural diet has been the transfer of viruses from one species to another.

BSE is a virus in cattle that attacks the brain and causes dementia, it is invariably fatal and it is closely related to sheep scrapie and the human brain disorder Creutzfeld Jakob disease. BSE is 'unusually resistant to heat and the normal sterilisation process'. The BSE virus will have entered the human food chain via milk and beef products (including beefburgers). It will, however, be several years before the effect on human health is known, as the virus lies dormant for long periods before the brain disease appears.

Even without the fear of BSE, the beefburger is high in salt and saturated fat, chemical flavourings, colourings and preservatives – it contains virtually no roughage. The beefburger is a recipe for heart attack, cancer, high blood pressure, obesity and constipation. Meanwhile the hygiene standards in 90 per cent of British slaughterhouses are so low that they are considered unfit to export meat to any other country.

Every minute 13,000 people worldwide eat identical products at well-known chain restaurants. The owners of the chain are not responding to consumer demand, on the contrary they are controlling the market. For every pound spent, five pence goes directly towards their advertising budget. Their beefburger is portrayed as a cheap, cheerful convenient food. Yet can anyone describe a tasteless burger in a 'rubber' bun as their ideal meal?

Rainforests – The burger chains are notorious for their involvement in the deforestation of the Amazonian rainforest. Enormous tracts of forest are cleared and the land is ranched for beef. In America it is impossible to prove where the burger chains' beef originates from, but it is widely believed that they are the major purchaser of Central American beef. They threaten legal proceedings against anyone daring to suggest they are responsible for rainforest destruction.

Dishonest – Burger chains have been the subject of court cases themselves – in Britain as a result of their abuse of child labour and in America for a dishonest advertising campaign which tried to promote their food as healthy! In the words of the Texas Attorney General: 'Their food is, as a whole, not nutritious. The intent and result of the current advertising campaign is to deceive customers into believing the opposite.'

Slaughter – The beef served in Britain's burger chains is largely domestically supplied – this is no reason to feel appeased. The suffering of the farm animal is immense; the cattle market, transportation to slaughter, and the slaughter process itself are a well-documented nightmare for these beautiful and docile animals.

'Humane' slaughter is a myth. A consultant pathologist writing in *Meat Magazine* (November 1986) described how the captive bolt method used to pre-stun cattle often doesn't work: 'It is a horrifying fact that approximately one third of the cattle shot in this way are not stunned, but stand grievously wounded and fully conscious while the pistol is reloaded.'

Now for a look at MILK. Human milk contains nine times less protein than cow's milk, yet has the best and highest concentration of amino acids. The body builders obtained from breast milk are of excellent quality. When the baby is weaned and put on to cow's milk, the infant is bombarded with nine times more protein than it needs, and problems like infantile eczema or asthma are common. The quality of protein is therefore very important. Less so is the quantity. With the help of amino acids – the building blocks of life composed of carbon, hydrogen, oxygen, nitrogen and sulphur – our protein intake will renew body tissue. We need cell renewers because life is a constant renewal of cell tissue. A high protein tissue selects the actual amino acid it needs. This does not, however, mean that we have to eat as much protein as possible as some people do in their ignorance of bodily functions and chemical processes.

We must, I repeat, take care not to go overboard. Protein is required for body repair and maintenance, and gives us energy, but there are detrimental effects if too much protein is ingested. For young children and some sportspeople a more-than-average protein intake is required to help the growth, development and strength of their muscles. However, extra exercise will also be of help in such cases and often a carbohydrate-rich diet will serve the athlete better. Again, we have to deal with people on an individual basis. I have been employed by various well-known football clubs as medical and nutritional adviser and have spoken to the players individually. Often it has been obvious that some players were in need of more protein than other players. On the whole, however, I have seen fit to introduce a diet higher in carbohydrates than in protein. At one time this advice caused me considerable problems with the wife of one of our best-known Scottish internationals. She was adamant that her husband needed protein and more protein. I asked her if she loved him and she replied, 'Of course!' I then advised her to make his salad plate larger and his meat plate smaller and she would stand a much better chance of keeping him. I am glad to say that we parted as friends.

A little more about dairy food is necessary here because I know that it causes much confusion. All milk is pasteurised nowadays and I will not for a moment dispute the wisdom of this. But unfortunately the pasteurisation process destroys the naturally occurring enzymes which help us to digest milk, thereby rendering it a much less valuable protein. Not so long ago we still had a choice. If we could afford it we chose to buy a bottle of milk with a gold top and this had a deep layer of rich cream at the top. If you didn't want the cream or couldn't afford it, you would buy your milk in bottles with a silver top – this had less cream. The cream rises to the top because it contains butterfat. When the fat rises to the top it comes into contact with the air and the oxygen combines with the fat on the top of the milk and turns it sour. One hundred years ago, this process did not pose so many problems. Most people lived near to a farm and the cities were very much smaller than nowadays. The farms reached into the suburbs of the cities, and it didn't take long for milk to travel from the cow to the consumer. The transportation and storage of milk wasn't a big problem. Half a century later things began to change and problems were experienced because the cities were growing larger and farms were being pushed out further into the countryside. Once the cows were milked, it was taking considerably longer before the milk reached the consumer. It was at this time that the commercial dairy industry began to be troubled with complaints about sour milk. The milk itself was no different. The complaints arose simply because in the natural process the fat rose to the top of the milk where it started combining with the oxygen in the air, turning the milk sour.

Then along came someone who claimed he could solve this problem: he had developed homogenisation. The butterfat rises to the top because it consists of small balls or globules of fat which are less dense than the rest of the milk; it is the law of nature that these float to the top. Homogenisation is a process in which the milk is filtered through a kind of screen. The milk passes through the filter without any problems, while the cream needs to be forced through the filter at high speed. This causes these small balls of cream to split and separate into very tiny balls of fat and the benefit is that when they are small enough they will not float to the top.

One of nature's mechanisms to help digestion of milk was not taken into account when this process was developed, however. Probably it was not understood. The little balls of fat which constitute the cream, it turns out, are surrounded by an enzyme that helps calves digest the fat. When this enzyme is ingested, the stomach starts the process of digesting the fat. Mostly, fat digestion in humans does not start until the fat reaches the upper intestine and is not finished off until the protein reaches the liver. This organ is designed to handle the digestion and the use of fat in our body. When you drink milk straight from the cow, the above process is followed, but when the milk is homogenised, the enzyme has been destroyed and the very tiny balls of fat are not recognised and will pass right through the upper intestine without being digested. This allows the fat to enter the body. When this fact was realised, it did not appear to be a problem. These tiny balls of fat would still eventually pass through the liver and become digested. The digestion process would still take place, only at a slightly later stage. The liver would filter and purify all the blood before it re-entered the circulation. Problems occur when these little balls of fat carry enzymes along with them. The main purpose of these enzymes, once they get inside an artery, is to eat and attack the inside of that artery. That appears to be their natural function. Once the enzyme gets into the liver, this organ will dispose of it. But the first time around the body it bypasses the liver and starts wreaking havoc in the arteries. It attacks and destroys the inner lining of the artery and particularly the inner lining of the heart and coronary arteries, which go back and forth between the heart and lungs.

Buttermilk, however, is something quite different. For a refreshing drink it can be mixed with an equal proportion of tomato juice; it can be served with a baked potato or as a salad dressing and is a source of excellent protein. Yoghurt is a rich source of bacteria able to synthesise some of the important factions of the vitamin B complex. It is also an excellent provider of good bowel bacteria.

An egg yolk, when used raw, contains good, natural lecithin. The problem is that during cooking or baking this lecithin is rendered useless.

As for cheese, also an excellent source of protein, I must stress that many cholesterol problems originate from cheese. Don't over-indulge in Cheddar cheese, which has a fat content of 80 per cent as opposed to the 40 per cent of Gouda or Edam cheese. The produce itself is a good protein source but is often spoiled by its high fat content and incompetence on behalf of the cheese producer or manufacturer who very often uses harmful colourings and additives. The most wonderful cheese to eat is the one that is made from warm milk in the natural, old-fashioned way. It does no harm to consider the origin of the cheese and, although the label may class it as 'all natural', it's often worth our while to question this assumption. An island cheese, or a cheese made on one of the smaller farms, is often more nutritious and healthy.

The best cheeses are made from raw milk during the months of spring when the grass is young, especially milk from cattle which have grazed on unfertilised pastures. I can highly recommend these, but unfortunately they are not common in Britain. In the United States and in the Netherlands they are popular and more widely available.

Now I want to come back to eggs briefly, because they can indeed be a good source of protein. Firstly, free-range eggs are by far the best. These are produced by hens that are raised naturally on the ground and allowed to scratch around at their leisure. Check the food used for the chickens as maize produces the best tasting eggs. If you are able to secure a good supply of free range eggs, treat yourself to a soft-boiled egg occasionally, but not more than three or four times a week at the most.

A high protein meal can cause insulin to peak or even hypoglycaemic levels to occur and it is worth remembering that vegans have the amino acids they need to function properly, even though they do not eat any animal or dairy protein. If we consider the diet of Eskimos only one or two generations ago, we find that the incidence of cancer was unknown, and according to our standards their dietary protein intake was very high, but it was harmless. The Maoris in traditional times had their diet worked out well and they experienced very little illness and disease. This has changed since the introduction of our dietary habits: they have not thrived since. Once they were the best dancers and the most ferocious fighters in the world; now, because of our 'polluted' diet, we have contributed to the loss of their inherited health.

I had a look at a Longevity Centre low-protein menu which was strictly vegetarian. I am sure that many dieticians would shrink from recommending it, but the resulting quality of life it would bring about would be marvellous.

Remember that a low protein diet is also a low stress diet and in this day and age that is of great value. Together with Alfred Vogel I formulated just such a low stress diet years ago. This we successfully introduced to patients in our clinic for natural and alternative therapies during the 1950s in the Netherlands. The diet is as follows:

Breakfast
Muesli mixed with the juice of an orange, grated apple, half a banana or other fruit. One or two pieces of Ryvita or wholemeal bread spread with natural vegetable margarine (sunflower or corn oil). One cup of tea after the meal, preferably peppermint, rosehip or chamomile. Bambu coffee may be used as an alternative.

Midday Meal
A plate of fresh vegetables, preferably containing carrot and beetroot. Also some raw and cooked vegetables. The fresh vegetables can be mixed with a sauce made from olive or sunflower oil with a little lemon or celery juice. Baked or steamed potatoes in their jackets may be taken with the vegetables. For dessert take yoghurt (low fat) with honey.

Evening Meal

Muesli, then fresh fruit salad. If you have a tendency to indigestion do not eat these together. Vegetable soup from vegetable remains, made with apple, radish, figs, leeks and tomatoes. Use salt sparingly – a little Herbamare salt is much better.

General

Animal fat is prohibited. Use eggs sparingly. No white flour, white sugar (or products made with them), pork, sausages, bacon or ham. Cut down, or even better avoid completely, coffee, alcohol, nicotine and sweets. Take enough outdoor exercise to obtain fresh air. Increased activity is recommended, e.g. cycling or walking instead of driving or being driven.

I am quite sure that many people would benefit from this diet and although protein is essential to life, it is also possible to lose life because of excess protein.

9

Carbohydrates

WHEN I TELL ladies at our slimming clinic that I prefer carbohydrates to proteins the look of horror on their faces is quite amusing. Their doubt and disbelief is obvious. Mostly I remind them that people on a high protein diet are often highly strung. Moreover, on a low carbohydrate diet, it is actually easier to lose weight. If the carbohydrates are from a good source, they are superb body builders.

Undoubtedly, SUGAR must be considered the major enemy to our health. Every day in the treatment of my patients, I am confronted by the effects of this substance. Do any of us ever think how many times daily we eat sugar-containing products or drink a sweetened beverage? There are so many hidden sugars in everyday food products that if we made an effort to count the spoonfuls of sugar we ingest each day, we would, in fact, be shocked. An elderly patient of mine put this to the test. She was unable to believe that her sugar intake was excessive, and she decided to jot down her entire sugar intake for a full day. When she multiplied this by seven to calculate her weekly intake, she realised that it was easier to measure her net monthly intake in bags rather than ounces. It appears that 88 lbs of sugar per capita is consumed each year in Britain. This is equivalent to approximately 40 bags of sugar. It seems that nothing is more addictive than sugar.

The power of advertising does nothing to assist in curbing people's sugar intake and children especially are an easy target for unscrupulous manufacturers. It is nearly impossible to keep children off sugar and I have come across many cases of hyperactive hypoglycaemia, all because there is too much sugar in children's diets. It is now widely acknowledged that sugar is the cause of many dental problems such as dental caries or the appearance of holes in the teeth. Unfortunately, it is a lesser-known fact that sugar has a similar effect on the bones. Whenever sugar touches the tongue it prevents the absorption of vitamins, minerals and trace elements. Even a partial reduction in sugar intake will be noticeable in one's health. Try cutting out sweets and snacks and look for a healthy alternative. It is true that sugar gives energy, but only in short bursts, and more sugar is needed each time. Sugar does not provide a sustaining energy.

The other day I enquired about a patient's daily intake of liquids. She proudly told me that she didn't take any sweet drinks and was surprised when we worked out the sugar intake from liquids alone. If we decide to choose sugar-free drinks this has to be a step in the right direction. Colas, fruit squash, fizzy lemonades and hot chocolate are all sugar-containing drinks. It would be much more beneficial to drink unsweetened tea or coffee, herb or fruit teas, low calorie drinks or water rather than these. Let's do our young children a favour and cut down their sugar intake. If they are not accustomed to too much sweetness, they will not have to learn to break a dangerous habit in later years, then they will be grateful to you.

Derek Cooper wrote an article in *Scotland on Sunday* on 4 August 1991 concerning the dangers of sugar. Everyone, he says, is in agreement that we eat far too much refined sugar for the good of our health. The hidden sugars are a major problem; it has been estimated that 70 per cent of the sugar we consume is contained in processed food, which fills the supermarket shelves. The sugar industry is not afraid to use dubious information in its advertising campaigns. Another excellent article, by Christine Doyle, appeared in the *Daily Telegraph* of Tuesday, 18 June 1991. We first spoke a few years ago, around the time my book *Neck and Back Problems* was published, and I told her then that many neck and back problems were caused by the wrong dietary management, including the consumption of too much sugar. In the article she quotes a recommended sugar intake not exceeding 10 per cent of the total daily calorie intake. At present up to 20 per cent of our calories is from sugar.

From a new report it was noted that where average sugar consumption was less than 60 grammes a day, tooth decay was rare. Whilst sugar is not thought to play any major role in the development of heart disease, the report points out that in certain individuals, high levels of added or hidden sugars may have undesirable metabolic effects. When I asked a heart specialist what he considered to be the greatest enemy to heart patients, he immediately replied 'Sugar'. Doubtless sugar causes cholesterol, glucose and insulin levels to rise. Read the frightening facts Christine Doyle compiled in the article mentioned under the heading 'Sugar Sums – Measured in Teaspoons':

Crunchie bar (six)

Aero (three and a half)

Packet of Polo mints (six)

Can of Coca-Cola (seven)

Glass of Ribena (six)

Glass of lemonade (two)

Chocolate digestive biscuit (two)

Two plain biscuits (half)

Bowl of Sultana Bran cereal (one)

Bowl of Coco Pops (three)

Doughnut (one and a half)

Instant Whip (ten)

Medium slice of fruit cake (three)

Small block of ice-cream (nine)

Small carton fruit yoghurt
(three)

Three teaspoons brown
sauce (one)

Three teaspoons Horlicks
(two)

Half medium tin baked
beans (two)

A great deal more sugar is eaten than is really needed. Over the last hundred years or so the consumption of sugar has grown, to the great alarm of health experts. People have become so addicted to sweet tastes that products that were never intended to contain any sugar have been given some anyhow to bring out their flavour.

As part of our carbohydrate intake, we need starchy foods as well as some sugars. I have seen people who could use their teeth like pliers even though they ate sugar and sugar-containing products. The difference is that they ate good quality sugar, such as raw cane or soft brown sugar, fruit sugar, or honey, for example, not the white refined sugar which is most harmful. We may need sugar for a quick burst of energy and occasionally a sugar product will not harm the body. It becomes dangerous, however, when sugar is used as a substitute for other foods, and the diet becomes less nutritious; it should never be used to replace fibrous foods which are essential for the digestive process. In cases of diabetes and hyperactivity, sugar must be treated with caution. I am involved in a research project, as I mentioned, which is aimed at defining and establishing a link between nutrition and character deviations. In cases of hyperactivity I have often seen the terrible consequences of an excessive sugar intake for children and those who have become prisoners.

Raw cane sugar and Demerara sugar may be used instead of refined white sugar as they are less harmful, but they have no nutritional value either. The sugar taken from cane as a thick black syrup is a better sweetener, but honey is the best sweetener of all. This source of energy contains minerals and trace elements, sucrose, fructose, along with certain enzymes. It is the lack of enzymes in processed sugar that makes it so difficult to digest.

Honey scores here again, because it is easily digested. The same is true of blackstrap molasses, which is a good form of sugar, being rich in minerals, enzymes and vitamin B complex. As for honey, a honeycomb is a most valuable source of unsaturated fatty acids. Used as a spread on toast or wholegrain bread, it is of tremendous value.

BREAD is a staple food product in our daily diet and, if it is of good quality, is a very dependable food. However, British health experts have said that our wheat lacks the vital mineral that helps prevent cancer and heart disease – selenium. In fact, most kinds of bread produced today do not have a single organically grown grain in them and therefore lack some of the minerals and trace elements which are so important for our health.

I would like to add a few more words on the subject of wheat, one of the main ingredients in bread. For a growing number of people wheat is becoming a threat as allergic reactions to the grain are now becoming more commonplace. Wheat should contain four chromosomes, but because of artificial administration during the process of growth, it may contain 60 or 70 chromosomes per grain. The human body cannot cope with this bombardment. Allergies result. I have lived with primitive people who eat more wheat than anybody in our part of the world. They have no allergic reactions to wheat, or gluten, however, because their wheat is from an organic source. The artificial processing of the wheat grain in soil that lacks minerals such as zinc, selenium, iron, calcium, etc., produces an imbalanced and one-sided source of food, lacking any nutritional value. True, the British soil is known to be poor in selenium and zinc; this seems to stem from the Ice Age when water from the melting icecap leached these minerals from the soil. Yet this does not change the fact that we should attempt to grow our wheat as naturally as possible. Make sure that the wheat you use has originated from good organic sources, otherwise wheat allergies may well occur. Unknown to many people, these can even become apparent in the skin.

Recently there has been an alarming increase in colitis and many allergic reactions to gluten have been diagnosed. Gluten allergies especially can lead to very serious problems such as multiple sclerosis. It is often the case that a gluten-free diet can bring about a major improvement in this degenerative condition. In my book on multiple sclerosis I have written in detail on the dangers of gluten and wheat. Gluten can cause the tissue in the small intestine to deteriorate, for example, as seen in celiac patients. Gluten, found in cooked wheat, flour and grains, can be released in a doughy mass and pose a real problem for the digestive process. The gluten protein may become a considerable obstacle to the working of protein digestive enzymes and the inefficient digestion of protein is likely to release peptin chains whose absorption is liable to fight the immunological system and can lead to allergic reactions.

Never ignore, then, what you think is a minor allergy, because if it is allowed to remain unchecked, it can lead eventually to a widespread degenerative condition. Protein foods such as bread, cakes and biscuits can cause or aggravate such allergies, because they can generate glucose flooding and inefficient protein digestion. But don't despair. Wheat can easily be avoided. Nature has been kind to us and supplies us with many alternatives, such as rye. Unfortunately, however, rye is a rather difficult grain to digest, and initially it may cause wind and flatulence, so as always chew well to allow plenty of saliva to mix with it. This is not the case with millet and I am delighted that millet is finally getting wider recognition. Millet is a well-balanced food source and has been recognised as such for centuries. The biblical prophet Ezekiel recorded the best laws ever given to man for food and hygiene, and millet was a recommended and established part of the diet. His advice on a balanced diet made millet into a life builder. Maize corn is also easier to digest and probably less dangerous than wheat.

For digestive purposes the right foods must be chosen and this is why rice is such an excellent product. Although generally it is classed as a carbohydrate, I would prefer to put it in a class of its own. To me it is neither a protein nor a carbohydrate food. It is a 'yin and yang' food that balances its carbohydrates and protein levels. And remember that brown rice is a great deal tastier than white rice; it has the added advantage that it does not go sticky.

Rice also contains fibre, vitamins and minerals, but it is important to cook the rice in the correct way to retain these. It's a food that is alive and in order to keep it alive, the method of cooking is important.

Put the desired quantity of rice into a casserole or ovenproof dish. Pour over boiling milk or, preferably, water. Have the oven pre-heated at the highest temperature, and place the dish of rice in the oven for ten to 15 minutes. Switch the oven off and leave the rice inside for five to six hours. Chop an assortment of vegetables, such as parsley, chicory, celery and cress, and mix through the rice with a little garlic salt. When required heat through.

It's reassuring to know that the world produces more rice than any other grain and that rice keeps excellently in shipping and storage when unpolished. Rice can be a good nourishing meal in itself, and it is so versatile that it can feature either in a main course or in puddings and desserts. It is highly nutritious and easily digested. Brown rice contains about 8 per cent protein of very good biological value and is about 79 per cent carbohydrate, chiefly starch. It has a tremendous supply of calcium, phosphorus, iron, copper traces, vitamins such as B1, B2, niacin and vitamin E. Its versatility means that it can play a major role in a healthy diet. I have been able to help many patients by introducing rice into their diet.

At the beginning of the chapter I said that carbohydrates are undesirable only when they are refined. Think of the carbohydrates in raw cereals, wholemeal bread, unpolished rice, and grains which have been grown in natural soil. These carbohydrates are of great benefit. Remember that wholegrains, such as rice, barley, wheat, rye, millet and buckwheat, have been part of the human diet since the Stone Age. For thousands of years the entire population of Japan has lived on a diet of rice, raw fish, land and sea vegetables and soya bean products and there is very little evidence of any degenerative disease there.

As a group, wholegrains are an excellent food, providing a good balance in carbohydrates, fats, fibre, protein and minerals. A meal of wholegrains will be digested slowly over a period of several hours, whereas the digestion of sugar and flour products takes only minutes. From wholegrains there is a slow and sustained release of glucose, which gently drifts into the bloodstream, to be used almost immediately by the muscles. There is no pressure on the pancreas to produce insulin, nor are there great demands on the liver. Grain fibre has a vital role to play in nutrition, but it is important to eat little and chew it well.

To appreciate the importance of this advice, the reader ought to be reminded that many conditions can be formed according to genetic information. Such information is carried by DNA via RNA, transformed into enzymes which control the body chemistry. Input of the right chemicals will deliver positive energy. Many physical and mental disorders have their root in the wrong body chemistry or metabolism. It's all too easy to say 'You'll have to live with it', but with some adjustment in our daily food pattern many conditions can be changed and sometimes even removed. Many distressing symptoms are no more than signs that the body wants to get rid of toxic material or that incorrect food is causing the metabolism to suffer. In previous chapters I have already mentioned the cause of certain liver and kidney complaints; many allergic conditions and twentieth-century diseases I would like to stress again, have been the result of the wrong dietary pattern.

Another staple food I would like to deal with is the POTATO. Nowadays it is sometimes said that the potato is a nightshade vegetable and cannot be good for anybody. Yet the potato, which is available on more or less a year-round basis, provides us with excellent means of reducing the acidity of the body. Raw potato juice is very effective in neutralising uric acid in rheumatic conditions, and also for combating stomach ulcers, eczema, psoriasis, duodenal ulcers and probably inflammation of the joints. When a potato is cooked in the skin, so that it maintains its properties, it is an excellent source of carbohydrate. If grown in good fertile soil the potato inherits the mineral qualities contained in the soil. It therefore becomes an outstanding food product. Often I also rely on its therapeutic properties in the treatment of my patients so that, despite the fact that potatoes generally are not greatly appreciated, I frequently advise patients to incorporate them in their diet.

I have already discussed the carbohydrate content of fruit and vegetables in the relevant chapter, but I haven't yet told you that dried fruits are very rich in potassium. As it may not always be possible to obtain a variety of fresh fruits, it's good to know that dried fruits also have healthy properties.

Here I would like to suggest to you that it makes good sense to have a starter of raw food before eating a main course of cooked food. It's true that not all nutritional experts agree on this, but I think the procedure helps combat the appetite more effectively and, because fresh food takes longer in digesting, gives more satisfaction. Raw food stills the initial hunger and also prevents over-eating. It also supplies us with extra enzymes for the digestion. If at all possible 50 per cent of our food should be eaten raw. For breakfast try a bowl of sliced or cubed fruit and later in the day some fibre. To increase the fibre content in any meal add some oat bran. This is very nutritional and also provides energy.

The nutritional quality of wholefoods and their content of vitamins and minerals is, as suggested, totally dependent upon the type of soil on which the produce was grown. As a member of the Soil Association I know how many rules there are to ensure the nutritional value of all agricultural produce. All the same, once crops have been harvested, especially vegetables and fruits, they immediately lose nearly 50 per cent of their original food value. If they were not raised in good soil in the first place, there will be even less food value left. Eating raw food means eating food in as near to its original condition as nature produced it.

It is obvious that one should not eat the skin of a banana, which is in place to protect the soft inner fruit, but we should eat the skin of a potato, an apple or a peach. Remember, I often prescribe carrot and beetroot as an integral part of natural therapies. The enzymes in raw foods are important, and so it is best to eat salads before cooked foods, thereby ensuring the body has a helpful supply of enzymes, minerals and trace elements. Carbohydrates can be our best friends and should be eaten in as wide a variety as possible when they are in season. As I have explained, eating a wide variety of foods is important for a number of reasons. Adjust your eating habits to suit your way of life and to achieve the best possible results. It was Adele Davis, who is an expert in the field of nutrition, who first suggested that it might be best to eat the biggest and healthiest protein meal in the morning. An experiment on yourself will provide the best proof of this.

Back in the Stone Age people ate berries and grains only when they were hungry, and they kept themselves healthy and fit. Nowadays we eat because we want to eat and in doing so we eat far too much. Social eating is an enjoyable pastime, but often we eat the wrong foods in an effort to please others. Now that the world seems to have become so much smaller, foods from other countries and cultures are easily available to all of us. In the West we can eat internationally, whether we feel like a Latin American meal, an Italian dish, or food from the Middle or Far East, for example. We can visit restaurants which specialise in certain types of cuisine. Failing that, we can find most of the necessary ingredients on the shelves of our local supermarket. Let me point out that it also works in reverse. In underdeveloped countries I have visited, the once healthy population is paying the price for eating food that is disagreeable to their digestive systems. On the whole it can be said that they stand to gain very little indeed from the way food is processed in the Western world and then exported. Nature designed man and his digestive system according to what was available in the environment where he lived. With our preparation methods we have caused much damage and placed under a great strain our digestive and absorption system. In doing so we have invited disease by failing to follow the rules of good nutrition.

Fruit of the season, sprinkled with some fibre or nuts, makes an excellent breakfast. Lunch is an ideal time for a good salad and the ingredients for a main meal can be decided upon according to the dietary advice in this book. Just think what can be done with a cabbage. It is a provider of first-class carbohydrates; raw cabbage mixed with grated carrot, a little honey and a few herbs provides us with a delicious and nutritious meal. By changing the types of herbs we can experiment with all kinds of different flavours. Interesting meals can be produced by anyone with a little imagination.

If you have a weight problem, make sure that your main meal is always eaten during the day, preferably at noon. It's better to have a large meal of salad, fruit or vegetables at night, as the body metabolism slows down after six o'clock in the evening; the digestive process can work away at this raw input and still leave one satisfied. Unfortunately, however, most people who are trying to lose weight manage well all day then yield to temptation and indulge in something sweet at night; they conveniently forget that sugar is an empty carbohydrate which has absolutely no food value. Problems result. Sometimes I say that the body contains one hundred trillion waste receptacles. Scientists have calculated that each person has somewhere between 70 and 100 trillion cells in the body – that means that one has over 70 trillion 'garbage cans' that need to be emptied. Proper food will mean proper detoxification. Effective detoxification is vital for the purity of the blood, whose existence ultimately depends on food that is ingested through the mouth. That food, along with oxygen, will eventually be transformed into energy, carbon dioxide, water and waste products. If the balance is good, it will leave the body and not become toxic and do damage. Such foods as white flour and white sugar – in fact all refined foods – are extremely hard on the liver and might have adverse effects. The liver will enjoy fresh wholegrains, which are easily digested.

How should one go about changing one's diet? It need not be done all at once. Start by eating only when you feel like eating, not when the clock says that it's time for a meal. Don't allow yourself to become fanatically obsessed about food or calories, and remember that you eat only for yourself and not for anyone else. Your natural intuition will tell you what is good or what is bad for you. Remember, the fresher the food the better it is for you. Carefully read the advice in the chapter on Food Combining. Quite often a person will feel better after only a minor change in diet. Take one step at a time. Instead of meat, try eating some more fish and see how much better you feel, or try changing a fruit breakfast to a more fibre-orientated breakfast. By experimenting you will soon know what is best for you.

In the chapter on proteins I gave you an example of a low protein diet and at the close of this chapter I will give you an example of a low carbohydrate diet, which many of my patients have used. There are no hard and fast rules and I would suggest that you try to find out what suits you best. If you are prepared to count the carbohydrate content of each meal, your objective should be to stay within a limit of 60 grammes daily. This may not be too easy in the beginning, but I'm sure that it will eventually be worth your while.

Sir Robert McCarrison wrote: 'The greatest single factor in the acquisition and maintenance of good health is perfectly constituted food.' This is emphatically the case and with all dietary approaches I feel it is important to keep this in mind. Hence, what follows is an example of an excellent low carbohydrate diet worked out by a dear friend of mine, Kitty Campion. I have used this diet with many of my patients., who have found it beneficial. Kitty Campion has given me her kind permission to incorporate the diet in this book.

Breakfast

Small orange or half grapefruit. Poached egg with two beef sausages (make sure the sausages contain no preservatives). Half a slice of wholemeal bread or other wholegrain bread, with one level teaspoon mayonnaise. Herbal or regular tea. Milk if desired. No sugar.

Morning Snack

One cup skimmed milk, quarter of a cup of creamed cottage cheese. If bran is required as a supplement to combat constipation, add one teaspoon of coarse bran, stirred into the cheese.

Lunch

Clear soup. Chicken or tuna fish salad. Use 4 oz of protein food, one teaspoon mayonnaise, and lettuce, chicory, celery, spring onions, sliced tomatoes in unlimited amounts. Any vegetable from approved list may be used. One slice of brown bread. One level teaspoon mayonnaise. Beverage of choice.

Afternoon booster

Half cup of plain yoghurt. If desired, coarse bran may be stirred in. Cheese, natural not processed (not cheese spread) – 1 oz on one small wholewheat cracker.

Dinner

Clear soup. 4 oz tomato juice. Steak or chops or beefburger or fish (¼ lb cooked weight). Approved vegetable, tossed salad, with vinegar and oil dressing, using oil allowance. Strawberries with little yoghurt. Beverage of own choice.

Evening Snack

Half cup of skimmed milk or plain yoghurt (bran addition optional in yoghurt). 1 oz of any leftover chicken, cheese, meat or fish, or 1 teaspoon of peanut or other nut butter on two brown rice crackers.

Your vegetables will be selected from the following list. Eat a daily minimum of two cups to a maximum of four cups.

Approved Vegetables

Vegetables marked with an asterisk are a good source of vitamin C, and are often rich in other nutritional values. Asparagus, avocado, beet greens*, broccoli*, Brussels sprouts, cabbage, celery, chard*, chicory*, collards*, cucumber, dandelion*, egg plant, endive, green pepper, green or wax beans, kale*, kohlrabi, leeks, lettuce, mushrooms, mustard*, radishes, sauerkraut, spinach*, string beans, summer squash, tomatoes, tomato juice, turnip greens*, watercress.

Approved Fruits

Take two servings of fruit daily in amounts listed. Those marked with an asterisk are good sources of vitamin C. Fresh, canned, cooked or frozen fruits may be used providing they are free from added sugar. Don't peel fresh fruit. Peelings are fibre sources. Apple (small), apple sauce (half a cup), apricots (fresh – two medium), banana (half – small), blackberries (one cup), blueberries (two-thirds of a cup), cantaloupe* (one-quarter of six-inch melon), cherries (10 large), cranberries (one cup), dates (two), figs (fresh – two large), figs (dried – one small), grapefruit* (half – small), grapefruit juice* (half cup), grapes (12 large), grape juice (quarter of cup), honeydew melon (one-eighth – medium), mango (one small), nectarine (one medium), orange* (one small), orange juice* (half cup), papaya (one-third – medium), peach (one medium), pear (one small), pineapple (half cup), pineapple juice (one-third cup), plums (two medium), prunes (two medium), raspberries (one cup), rhubarb (one cup), strawberries* (one cup), tangerine (one medium), water melon (one cup).

> NB: All fruits and vegetables, whether served cooked or uncooked, peeled or unpeeled, should be thoroughly washed before consumption. Pesticide residues help no one and can be reduced significantly by washing.

Protein substitutions may be made if desired. A quarter cup of cottage cheese may be substituted for one ounce of meat. Approximately two ounces of raw meat may be replaced with one egg. One ounce of Cheddar or any other hard cheese can replace about two ounces of meat, raw weight. Peanut butter is a good source of both protein and carbohydrates, but the commercial varieties contain saturated fat. Even if it's one of your favourite snack foods, eat no more than one tablespoon of peanut butter a week.

Supplements to Reducing Diet

Use one mega-multi-vitamin tablet together with one vitamin B complex tablet, both to be taken at breakfast.

Bran is more effective in the coarse than the finely ground form. Either form can be obtained in tablets as well as loose. Bran is not only useful for its laxative effects, but for suppressing the appetite and for helping weight loss. If you've never tried bran in your diet before, introduce it into your meals using only one teaspoon at a time. More than this may cause discomfort or flatulence. Aim to increase your bran intake until you are eating two tablespoons a day.

10

Food Combining

THE SO-CALLED 'Hay Diet' has deservedly been resurrected after being out of the limelight for a good many years and I couldn't be more pleased. The excellent book *Food Combining for Health*, written by Doris Grant and Jean Joyce, has given the old dietary system a renewed lease of life with its efforts to explain to its readers the advantages of this dietary plan. The tremendous interest from the public and the resulting publicity have further encouraged its wider acceptance and there now appears little or no controversy about the benefits of the system.

Dr Hay was born in 1866 in the United States of America, and considering the scarce nutritional knowledge available when he was around, he was well ahead of his contemporaries in his specialised field. Yet the kind of dietary system he devised is today much more necessary than it ever was in his day. The list of allergies and problems resulting from incorrect diets seems to grow ever longer, and in my work all too often I come across the results of poor digestion and absorption. These are good enough reasons to concentrate for a while on Dr Hay's work and the principles of food combining. Despite the many books devoted to such principles, there still remains considerable confusion surrounding them and therefore I have decided to include a section on food combining in this book. In today's hurried and stressful life one should pay more attention to them and in order not to confuse matters I will keep to the main points. Dr Hay also kept it simple. He had few rules, but his whole belief rested on a few major principles:

- Do not eat starches and sugars in the same meal
- Eat proteins, starches and fats only in small quantities
- Eat wholegrains and unprocessed foods in preference to these
- Banish refined sugars and refined flour from the diet
- Vegetables, salads and fruit must form a major part of the diet.

Well there you have it in a nutshell – the pillars upon which Dr Hay's diet was built. These points all seem quite sensible, but at the time it was produced his plan seemed revolutionary in its setting out of the principles of food combining! The major assertion of his dietary plan is that certain foods cannot be successfully combined as certain combinations place the digestive system under strain. Intervals of at least four to four and a half hours should be allowed between meals of a different type.

Food combining makes sense. Good digestion of our food is terribly important. Consider a serious disease such as cancer. So often I have thought that poor digestion and therefore ineffective absorption was the cause. With poor digestion, the body starts to lack vitamins, minerals and trace elements, and because of insufficient cell renewal the body degenerates. The constant chemical activity in the digestive system becomes ineffective and it has no control over what enters through the mouth. If our food intake is inadequate, problems will thus arise.

Starchy food needs a good alkaline digestive system, while proteins need an acid system for proper digestion and hydrochloric acid must be present for the chemical process to go ahead unhindered. With a little background information it becomes easier to understand how important the acid/alkaline balance is to one's general health. When this system fails, food which has only been partly digested begins to ferment in the stomach. If you would like this put in plain English, it actually starts to rot while it is still in the stomach. This presents ideal conditions for such dreaded diseases as cancer or *Candida albicans*. It represents the sort of situation in which a yeast parasite really feels at home and, of course, thrives. Poisonous waste material begins to attack the body, and the chemical machinery of the body will go from bad to worse. Once you have taken all this into account, sensible food combining sounds essential and it does not require any great mathematical knowledge. Even if only the major rules of food combining were to be followed, it would be a good start, especially since it is now widely believed that one of the major causes of degenerative disease is the mixing of proteins and starches.

Fruits are not easily combined with proteins, and neither do fruits combine too well with starches. It is sad that fruits and vegetables are often mixed, because they serve different purposes. Fruits set about cleaning up the chemical machinery of the body, while vegetables are body builders. Acid fruits do not combine well with sweet fruits and for that matter neither do many fruits combine well together. It is wiser to eat fruits separately and to try and eat fruits when they are in season.

Starches and sugars should not be eaten with proteins or acid foods. To reiterate, because I have seen so many patients with problems resulting from the use of white flour and white sugar, I cannot see any sense in using these. The refining process has removed whatever nutritional value these products had in the first place.

A proper acid/alkaline balance is very important and it is worth remembering in this context that fruit and vegetables are good alkaline foods.

Food combining is also a good way of reducing weight.

Following its principles many people hesitate about the wisdom of eating a dessert. According to its laws, it is always better for fruit to be eaten before a main meal and not after. The digestive system has an important task to perform when a main meal is eaten and certain fruits are not easily digested, especially not when eaten at the close of the meal. This would only hamper the digestion process.

Do not, by the way, drink too much liquid with a meal, as the idea of flushing one's food away is very poor. Saliva is the best digestant possible and food mixed with one's saliva will ensure proper digestion and will certainly be of benefit to the body.

Many people nowadays struggle to control the effects of wind, whether it be through burping or through flatulence in the stomach. These are signs that the body cannot cope with what we put into it and our digestion requires some well-deserved help. Always try to eat moderately. We overeat far too often, and the result is obesity, which doesn't do anyone's health any good. Food should be eaten with discipline and respect. Do not attempt to eat food that is too hot or too cold.

Diluted food or juices should always have preference over concentrated foods. There are many charts and books in circulation dealing with bad and good combinations and therefore I will not go into much detail. If you would like to go into the subject in more depth, you can easily obtain a publication which deals exclusively with food combining. Whenever physical problems occur, patients tend to become alarmed, and certainly even the smallest allergy deserves to be noted and investigated. In my book *Viruses, Allergies and the Immune System* I have given plenty of examples of possible causes and warning signals which were allowed to go unheeded. It is fun to have a healthy diet because one feels so much better and more energetic. The resulting weight loss and the increased energy feel like a new lease of life has been granted, and many times I have heard people wish that they had known about the benefits years ago. Even the older generation often express their appreciation and regret for not having made changes long before.

It is considered better to eat one's main meal during the day and not to eat much during the evening, after six o'clock. It is well known that the metabolism starts to slow down as the day progresses and it should not be overtaxed by expecting the digestive system to work overtime. It is better to spread food intake evenly over the day and this will keep hunger pangs away. Especially during mid-morning, one tends to look for something to eat – a piece of fruit would be the best choice here.

It is actually quite a good idea to eat fruit for breakfast as well as for a mid-morning snack. Then at lunchtime one can eat starch or carbohydrate food. A simple and light mid-afternoon snack can then be followed by an evening meal which can be more protein-orientated. These are quite simple guidelines and yet they are full of common sense. I know only too well from personal experience that on my travels such guidelines can be difficult to adhere to and it is always a relief to be home again, where it is easier to eat sensibly. At home I can manage much better not to give in to temptation. Frequent crossing of time zones and eating out in restaurants and living in hotels plays havoc with the digestion of most people. This is a fairly regular complaint, unless one happens to be very disciplined. The other day, sitting in the dining-room of a hotel abroad, I watched a person seated at a nearby table , who was indulging in a meal which contained at least three concentrated proteins. One's health is reflected in the whole body, and this person certainly looked a picture of discomfort with his very flushed complexion. In particular, be careful with fats, especially as they are likely to inhibit the secretion of gastric juices, and the chemistry of the body will then not work properly.

On every diet sheet that I work out for my patients, I state that at least once a day a salad of some sort must be eaten. This is indeed important. Fortunately, salad ingredients combine excellently with proteins and starches; for salad dressing use some

Molkosan (a whey product from the Bioforce range). Molkosan is often described as a milk-serum and for many years it has played a large part in traditional folk medicine in Switzerland and Germany. Indeed, during the nineteenth century, at least once a year wealthy society people used to make a trip to Switzerland to partake in the Swiss Whey Cure. It is an excellent product that ought to feature in all weight-reducing diets and it tastes very refreshing on a salad. On sale nowadays as formulated by Alfred Vogel many years ago, Molkosan contains many minerals, and as a concentrated liquid it is excellent, balancing alkalinity and acidity.

The body is a wonderful and technically faultless piece of equipment that will emit signals when something is wrong. The problem lies in whether we are able to interpret these signals correctly or not. In the case of wind, flatulence, or if the taste of food repeats itself with regularity, the body is trying to tell us either that the digestive process is being overworked, or that the mix of nutrients was incorrect. We then must look at acidity in the diet, because very often the cause can be found here. The bulk of each meal should consist of alkaline foods. With arthritis and rheumatic patients in particular, I first of all look for signs of excess acidity in the system and I have never yet failed to improve such conditions by advising correct food combining. Rheumatism, arthritis, duodenal and peptic ulcers, eczema and psoriasis are all born in an over-acid system and if the patient is prepared to co-operate, these problems can be reduced to a large extent by introducing a good alkaline and acid balance in the diet.

During my last American tour I met up again with a friend of long standing, Edward Alexanian. He has designed an excellent and extremely easy to follow food combining chart for efficient digestion and has worked and researched in this field for many years, all the while improving his theories. He has put together some very interesting material and has kindly allowed me to use his chart in this book, for which I am very grateful.

There is much to say on this particular subject and there are many publications available, but I reiterate one final piece of advice. Do not ridicule it as being too simple. Chew your food thoroughly. Juices are becoming more and more popular and there are many excellent vegetable and fruit juices, but my only reservation with juices is that from Creation we have been fitted with teeth that are capable of grinding and chewing our food, and teeth should be used. Raw foods are very good for the digestion and they serve to keep our bowels in good shape. The digestive system demands care and it should be remembered that what is imported should again be exported within 24 hours, or else we become constipated. I well remember the time that Alfred Vogel and I opened the first clinic for natural medicine in the Netherlands. Under the guidance of a medical professor we had an apparatus built specifically for upper bowel cleansing. I will never forget the time when the first patient underwent this treatment. The treatment involved approximately 30 pints of chamomile water being flushed through the bowels, and we were absolutely astonished at the quantity of waste material consequently disposed of. I doubt if any of us has any idea how much waste material is contained in the body of the average person, and we must agree that this is not a pleasant thought. This waste material must be disposed of, or else it encourages illness and disease. A good diet will result in good digestion and there will be no need for any unusual bowel cleansing treatment, although this can never do any harm. The aim should be to encourage the body to do it on its own. With a correct diet and 'lively' food, one can expect better health and more energy.

For easy guidance, please consult the following lists detailing which foods are alkaline or acid-based. This should enable you to plan your diet correctly and to choose the right nutrients for food combining.

FOOD COMBINING CHART FOR MORE EFFICIENT DIGESTION

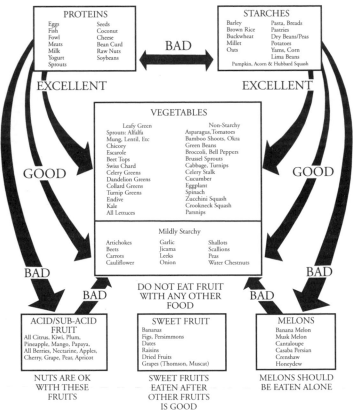

ACID/ALKALINE CHART – WHAT IS ACID AND WHAT IS ALKALINE? (opposite page)

The Alkaline/Acid balance of the body is 80 per cent to 20 per cent. Maintain the same balance in each meal.

Alkaline Vegetables
Alfalfa
Artichokes – both
Asparagus
Bamboo shoots
Beans – green, string
Beets – all
Broccoli
Cabbage – all
Carrots
Celery
Cauliflower
Chicory
Coconut – dried
Corn
Cucumber

Dill
Dulse
Endive
Garlic
Horse Radish
Kale
Leek
Lettuce
Mushrooms
Onions
Parsley
Parsnips
Peppers – sweet
Potatoes
Pumpkin
Radish

Sauerkraut
Soya Beans
Spinach
Sprouts
Squash
Turnips
Watercress

Acid Vegetables
Asparagus tips –
  white
Beans – all dried
Brussels sprouts
Lentils
Rhubarb

Alkaline Fruits
Apples & Cider
Apricots
Avocados
Bananas
Berries – all
Cherries
Currants
Dates
Figs
Grapes
*Grapefruit
*Lemons
Olives – sun dried
*Oranges
Peaches
Pears
Pineapple – fresh
Plums
Pomegranates
Prunes
Raisins
Tangerines
Tomatoes

Alkaline Dairy
  Produce
Yoghurt
Acidolphilus
  buttermilk
Milk – raw (human,
  cow or goat)
Whey

Acid Dairy Produce
Butter
Cheese – all
Cottage cheese
Cream
Custards
Milk – boiled,
  cooked, malted,
  dried, canned

Alkaline Nuts
Almonds
Chestnuts – roasted
Coconuts – fresh

Acid Nuts
All nuts not above
Coconut – dried

Alkaline Cereals
None

Acid Cereals
All flour products
All grains

Alkaline Flesh
  Foods
Blood & Bone only
Bonemeal

Acid Flesh Foods
All meat
Fish
Fowl
Gelatin

Alkaline Miscel
Agar
Coffee substitute
Honey
Kelp
Tea – China & Herb

Acid Miscel
Alcoholic drinks
Cocoa
Coffee
Condiments – all
Drugs
Eggs
Flavourings
Mayonnaise
Tobacco
Vinegar
Lack of sleep
Tea – Indian

Acid Fruits
All preserved fruit
Canned – sugared
Cranberries
Dried – sulphured
Glazed fruit
Olives – pickled

This chart shows the acid/alkaline forming foods. Foods marked * eat alone.

PROTEIN CHART

The food portions in this chart are based on 100 grammes or 3½ ounces. For example, 100 grammes of plain yoghurt gives 8 grammes of complete protein.

Complete Proteins

Skimmed Milk 1 Quart	35 Grammes
Torula Yeast	34 Grammes
Soya beans, cooked	30 Grammes
Swiss Cheese	28 Grammes
Cottage Cheese	19 Grammes
2 Eggs	13 Grammes
Yoghurt, plain	8 Grammes
Fish, boiled	25–30 Grammes

Complete Protein Combinations

Legumes and Brown Rice	24 Grammes
Sesame Seeds and Brown Rice	21 Grammes
Porridge Oats and Millet	15 Grammes
Beans and Corn	14 Grammes

FOOD COMBINATIONS

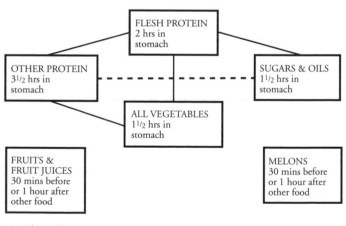

Avoid combining unjoined boxes
Boxes joined · · · · · combined okay
Boxes joined ———— combined excellently

11

Vitamins, Minerals and Trace Elements

VITAMINS PLAY A tremendously important role in nutrition and therefore in life. Recently, on one of my American trips, I visited a major health food store in Virginia. An elderly lady asked to see me. She started to talk, assuring me that she had no specific health complaints, but she wanted confirmation of her good health. I was impressed with the glint in her eyes, and although she was elderly, I soon realised that she was completely in tune with the times and 'with it'. She seemed to take a great interest in life and she was extremely fit. I discovered that she listened to music every day, played the organ during church services, had an important function in the Red Cross, and was chairwoman of several clubs. After all this she asked me how old I thought she was. I guessed that she was approaching 80. She told me, however, that she was in her 101st year. I looked at her in astonishment and she showed me some photographs and proof of her statement. I learned that she was a regular visitor to the health food store where we met, and she was delighted that the staff advised her on what she should or shouldn't eat. Over the years she had learned quite a bit about health, nutrition and immunity, and she proudly acknowledged that she knew that the body is made up of billions of cells, and that with every tick of the clock hundreds of them die. She knew good nutrition is needed for good health. A well-balanced and nutritious diet is essential. If our diet is inadequate it may be supplemented with vitamins, minerals and trace elements. Vitamins are part of all life processes and if a vitamin deficiency were to arise for any reason, we would not be able to function correctly. The old lady had functioned well all her life. She had taken care of her diet and she still had her own teeth and did not use glasses. Because she had invested in life, now in her advanced age she was reaping the benefits.

Older generations often knew by instinct or by tradition that certain foods would help to prevent disease. In 1910 a little more knowledge was gained about foods using scientific tests. In all, 13 different vitamins were isolated from various foods and ever since then, nutrition and the role of vitamins has been a much studied subject. The conclusions reached as a result can often make depressing reading. If we look at processing with its many additives, or the irradiation of food, it is a simple matter to conclude that there can be very few vitamins, minerals and trace elements left in our list. Too often we have seen during famines in the Third World that, when food and nutrition is inadequate, illness and disease result from deficiencies. It is astonishing that even in this day and age, with all our knowledge of nutrition, I occasionally see scurvy or pellagra caused by vitamin deficiencies.

Teenagers are particularly at risk. It is not uncommon for teenagers nowadays to lack the correct food during their years of rapid growth, because their diet contains such a large amount of junk food. Such foods are body breakers rather than body builders, and their repeated intake means that the demands of the growth process cannot be met nutritionally. During this time, girls especially become aware of their waistlines and they cut their calorie intake to reduce weight. Unfortunately, they usually cut out the foods they need most, resulting in an inadequate diet and the production of an ideal breeding ground for health problems.

It is distressing to see babies arrive in this world already inflicted with degenerative disease. Sadly, this is happening more often. Either the condition is inherited or the mother's diet during pregnancy was inadequate and lacked vitamins, minerals and trace elements. While in the uterus, the baby uses whatever is available and feeds off the mother like a parasite. In other words, it takes all the nourishment it needs from the mother, often leaving the mother depleted. If the mother does not have a sufficiently good diet to start with, the baby cannot acquire the correct mix of ingredients for healthy growth. Some babies, as a result, have been born with arthritic conditions, for example, which in later life may become more pronounced and result in congenital degenerative disease. During pregnancy women are responsible for themselves as well as their unborn babies, which is all the more reason to eat wisely and well.

The metabolism slows as we get older, perhaps because the body requires less energy. Elderly people often lose their appetite and pay less attention to having a good, wholesome diet. Mostly they won't even consider taking a vitamin supplement. If you are in this situation, please seek advice. Visit your local health food store where they will be happy to advise you.

Dieters, heavy drinkers, smokers, and even women who take the contraceptive pill, all have special dietary needs, hence the guidance in this book. Does our food contain all the ingredients necessary to keep the chemical industry of our body going? If you are in doubt, do something about it now. Don't wait until the signs are obvious. Nowadays it is so easy to bring in a takeaway or to have a frozen ready-made meal heated up in the microwave. We may be busy, but we are not doing ourselves any favours by eating such meals, because we need 'live' food to keep our energy levels topped up.

Until the age of industrialisation and automation people needed more energy in order to keep up their strength for the higher physical demands of their work. Although most employment is probably physically less demanding today, we work under stressful conditions, and stress can rob us of vitamins, minerals and trace elements. It is a fact that when a person is under stress the potassium level, for example, is depleted. Remember that it is in wholesome food, in fresh vegetables and fresh fruit, that vitamins, minerals and trace elements are found, and not in processed or pre-packaged food.

As I have said all too often, essential requirements are absent from our food right from its origin, because of the way our food is grown. The soil needs plenty of minerals such as calcium, iron, selenium and magnesium, if these nutrients are to be passed on into our food. Wholesome and nutritious food cannot be grown if the soil is lacking in minerals. If you are in any doubt, consider a vitamin supplement. A balanced multi-vitamin supplement such as Health Insurance Plus from Nature's Best follows the principle of a balanced diet and therefore is a really effective investment. One or two tablets a day is quite sufficient as they contain all the necessary minerals and trace elements.

As food nutrients sometimes interact, it makes sense to use a multi-vitamin. For instance, vitamin C is necessary for iron absorption, vitamin E improves the absorption of vitamin A, and zinc is necessary for the proper digestion of the vitamin A which is stored in the liver. Together with the other vitamins a multi-vitamin will maintain a good dietary balance. During the wintertime, periods of stress, long working hours, and situations which cause irregular meals, a good multi-vitamin becomes a necessity.

The therapeutic benefits of vitamins, minerals and trace elements can be easily proved in countries where the supply and quality of food is inadequate, thereby causing deficiency disease. In our part of the world, where we are fortunate enough to have sufficient food and plenty of choice, please let our choice be good food. Let it be food that has life in it.

Vitamin C deficiencies are becoming more commonplace and, especially during the winter months with the increased risk of colds and flu, vitamin C is vitally important as a stimulant for the immune system. I don't doubt that many twentieth-century diseases can be attributed to deficiencies. The immune system is a subject about which there is still much to learn, but it is known that it will respond quickly to a good diet. If problems have been recognised and the immune system needs extra help, try the supplement Michaels Quick Immune Response. I have worked with this formula for quite some time now and during my 30 years in practice I have changed and adapted it according to circumstances and requirements. During these years I have identified some of the factors that render the immune system less effective and I have designed this formula with the rebuilding of the immune system in mind. Nature's Best produce this supplement and if you want to avoid illness or disease, it will give the immune system a little boost or an extra bit of help to strengthen your resistance.

Nutritional supplements are becoming more important in today's world, as the basic requirements for good health – air, water and food – are deteriorating in quality. We have read plenty about food, but we should remind ourselves that both our water and air supplies are affected by environmental pollution. We have never been exposed to such harmful pollution in fact. Therefore we should protect ourselves with good food and supplementary vitamins, minerals and trace elements, as these ingredients are our only defence against environmental attacks. The battle for health can sometimes seem a hard one. It is remarkable what we come up against in, for example, the many side effects of additives, colourings, pesticides and so on. We will not be able to overcome the obstacles these represent if we persist in eating junk food, in using a microwave oven because it is so handy, or buying food that has been irradiated. Doing so at best renders our food lifeless, and what might have been healthy food to start with will lose all its character and benefits. This is a responsibility we must all deal with, but I still maintain that with a positive attitude we will be able to stand up to environmental attacks. We have little choice!

The body is sensitive and uses all kinds of alarm bells to forewarn us of an impending problem. A headache may be a first indication of poor diet or we may experience circulation problems. Dandruff may indicate that there is a lack of selenium, zinc, vitamin C and vitamin B6 and essential fatty acids. A digestive problem may mean that there is not enough folic acid, iron or niacin in the diet. Significant indicators are hair and nails, and any change here may tell us that there is not enough calcium, iron or copper in our system. If you feel that your sense of taste or smell has become impaired, this could be because of an inadequate zinc supply in the body. Osteoporosis has reached almost epidemic proportions because of lack of calcium, magnesium and zinc. Allergies, those tremendous modern-day problems, are mostly due to a lack of vitamins C, A and B complex. And so I could go on. The list is never ending. And it seems to grow all the time. Let's use some common sense and try to overcome these problems. I understand that there is much confusion on the subject of vitamins, but I have been consistent in my advice and have always advocated, where necessary, the use of supplementary vitamins, minerals and trace elements, and the necessity of a balanced diet.

A vast amount of research has been carried out and is still ongoing on the subject of food and nutrition. It is impossible to recommend a required daily intake; the best one can do is to recommend guidelines. With respect to essential fatty acids, I cannot resist using this opportunity to stress once again the benefits of the oil of evening primrose. I have already mentioned this product in the chapter on Fats and Oils and have drawn your attention to how much this is needed by the body. I have seen in my patients how successful it is in overcoming deficiencies.

One specific food product that is persistently lacking nowadays is lecithin. The technical name for this is a phospholipid, which is a complex mixture of choline, inositol, essential fatty acids and phosphorus. It is one of the richest natural sources of two important nutrients, choline and inositol. These two lipotropic agents play an important role in fat metabolism in the liver and the emulsification of fats in the body. Choline is a precursor, acetylcholine, a brain chemical concerned with passing messages between brain cells. For young people, or people whose work requires concentration, this nutrient is of great benefit, and Nature's Best produces several suitable supplements containing it.

Be sensible and look at what might be lacking in your body or diet. Think of what mineral nutrition is lost in the cooking process of foods; vitamins, minerals and trace elements are far more efficiently absorbed when bound up in food than when taken on their own. The body needs more than 15 different minerals for growth and energy, and minerals such as phosphorus, cobalt and zinc are needed to maintain the chemical processes of our body in good working order. Bear in mind the body cells and body fluids are highly dependent upon minerals.

Earlier I mentioned that when vegetables have been cooked, the cooking liquid is often then poured down the drain along with most of the goodness. Yet many of the people who do this are sufficiently concerned about their health to rush to the chemist or the health food store to buy vitamin supplements. I wonder if this is always necessary. If we eat food that has been grown with care, or grown organically, the need for supplements is unlikely. If we have problems obtaining organic food, we may well require supplementary vitamins, minerals and trace elements. These will help us to restore balance in our diet and give us the energy we need to cope with today's fast-moving lifestyle.

The following overview will give the reader at a glance information detailing from which source a specific vitamin is available, when to use it, and those most likely to require it.

Vitamin A   Milk, butter, eggs, liver
   For eyesight and mucous membranes

For toddlers and young children, pregnant women, dieters, sick people

Vitamin B1   Meat, grains, poultry
Tiredness, painful leg muscles, nervous system

Teenagers, older generation, dieters, sick people

Vitamin B2   Green vegetables, grains, meat, eggs, milk,
                 cheese
Deficiency causes skin problems

Teenagers, elderly generation, dieters, sick people

Vitamin B6   Green vegetables, grains, bananas, lean meat
Menstruation problems, blood, nervous system

Teenagers, pregnant women, elderly generation, users of the contraceptive pill, dieters, sick people

Vitamin B12   Milk, eggs, meat, fish
Maintenance and production of blood

Teenagers, elderly generation, dieters, sick people

Vitamin C   Citrus fruit, kiwifruit, cabbage, tomatoes,
                potatoes
Production of red blood corpuscles, tissue, bones, teeth; immune system

Teenagers, pregnant women, elderly generation, dieters, smokers, sick people

Vitamin D   Margarine, egg yolks, tuna, salmon
Deficiency causes weakness of the bones and poor teeth

Babies, toddlers and young children, elderly generation, sick people

Vitamin E   Grains, vegetables, vegetable oils and nuts
Tiredness

Everyone

Vitamin F   Milk, vegetables, egg yolks
Essential for the skin

Everyone

Vitamin K   Green vegetables
Resistance

Everyone

NB: All B vitamins improve the quality of the skin, gloss the hair and strengthen the nails.

12

Preservatives

THERE ARE THREE S's that I have come to regard as enemies to human health. These three S's will need to be exorcised somehow if we want to improve our health.

The first S stands for SALT. I sometimes wish that we could turn back the clock to when salt was first discovered. Long ago salt was a rare commodity. Traditionally, when one was invited to a feast, one sat either above the salt or below the salt. Those who sat above were allowed to partake of the salt. Those below were of a lower social order and were allowed no salt on their food. How I wish that salt was still a rare commodity and that its detrimental effects on health were recognised. Mostly salt is added during the preparation of food, yet many people still liberally shake the salt cellar over the food on their plate. Salt (or sodium chloride) indeed serves as a preservative, but it is also widely used as an extra treat for our taste buds. This is not at all sensible because we also know that salt retains fluid in the body and to people with a tendency to high blood pressure, it can actually be fatal.

An average person eats about 13 grammes – two and a half teaspoons – of salt a day. Two-thirds of this is added to products by the food manufacturer, as permitted by the Food Processing Act. The rest is added during cooking or at the table. We certainly need salt, but not too much. Alfred Vogel and I once visited a group of people who had no salt intake at all. We discussed this and expressed our surprise, but then we saw that every day they ate a certain bulb, as we eat potatoes or bread. That bulb, *Harpagophytum* – Devil's Claw – contained all the mineral salts these people needed.

All of us need some form of salt but up to three grammes – half a teaspoon – a day should be sufficient. One only needs to look at the rise in heart disease, kidney problems and strokes to understand why I am shocked at the level of our salt intake. Please, try seriously to use less salt when cooking, and avoid adding extra salt when the food is on your plate. It's better to use a salt substitute, of which many exist. Such substitutes or any other good alternative natural flavouring will enhance the flavour of your food equally well and possibly even better.

Unnecessary salt is added particularly to chips and snack foods – try to avoid this. When buying food check the labels carefully to see what is said about added salt. When making soup, please don't use too much salt or salted meat. The number of Asian people with high blood pressure who consult me is shocking. I have concluded that this is most likely because of their use of soy sauce, which contains monosodium glutamate. Packaged food, such as tinned and packet soups, also contain a lot of salt.

If we try to reduce our intake of salt slowly, however, we will not miss it, and eventually we will discover that we can quite easily do without it; this will also help to keep our weight under control. The main reason for reducing our intake, however, is that it will be better for our health. It is a feeble excuse that salt is needed for its minerals. Sure, salt contains some minerals, but the best sources of minerals are fruit and vegetables. Salt is a health destroyer and in the United States it is said that the cause of death can often be directly accredited to excessive salt intake.

Salt definitely has a drying effect on the body and moreover it is a deadly, inorganic substance which contains very little goodness. It destroys the calcium in the body and instead of giving our taste buds a treat, it apparently paralyses 260 taste buds in the mouth. When salt breaks down into sodium chloride, it becomes like a poison: the body decides naturally that it's necessary to wash the poisons from the stomach which arrive there via the kidneys. Aware of my own weakness for salt at one stage, I can't stress strongly enough the need to reduce our salt intake or banish it from the diet altogether. Man is a creature of habit and habits are difficult to break, but never impossible.

As a salt substitute try Alfred Vogel's sea salt, Herbamare. It is a delicious sea salt with a distinctive flavour, and its use results in extra-exciting meals. Herbamare is mineral-rich and contains 14 fresh herbs. For a somewhat more spicy taste try Herbamare Spicy, a similar seasoning but with the addition of red peppers. Both are ideal to liven up the simplest fare and have proven extremely popular. Alfred Vogel has always put great emphasis on a restricted and sensible salt intake. It's very difficult to make a nice sauce if salt is not permitted. By using a little sea salt one will not come to much harm. Unfortunately, there are those who see health-conscious nutrition as dull and flavourless, when in fact, with some of the products named, the opposite is the truth. Because of the range of seasonings and the variety of flavours which can be obtained, these products allow for exciting culinary adventures.

So, there is a choice of excellent substitutes which can be used in cooking for a reduced salt diet, with the big advantage that the taste and flavour liked by everyone will be preserved. Taking things with a pinch of salt is terribly important, but let this indeed be no more than a pinch, because then our health will benefit. Stop sprinkling salt liberally on food and use much less of it in cooking. Salt is sodium chloride and although a little sodium is essential for health, on average one eats about 20 times the amount needed. Excess salt intake is one of the main reasons why hypertension has become prevalent. Patients with hypertension should, in fact, be cautious with any food that contains sodium. This might prove difficult at first since it is included in so many products and is also part of the infamous monosodium glutamate. But start reducing your salt intake now, as it takes quite a while to rid the body of the toxic poisons caused by salt.

The second S stands for SUGAR. In the chapter on Carbohydrates I have already mentioned this substance, but I have more to add. Refined sugar, often used in preservatives, is a health hazard and to my mind it must be considered the second biggest health enemy behind salt. Refined sugar leads to an increase in the blood sugar level, causes stress and hyperactivity and whenever it touches the tongue, it starts to deplete the reserves of vitamins, minerals and trace elements in the body. Consider the damage it causes to teeth. Unfortunately, virtually all junk foods contain sugar. High cholesterol and over-stimulation of insulin, which might result from such products, are major contributory factors to diabetes. Sugar will also affect us mentally and excessive sugar intake may indeed instigate mental illness: who wants to make life a slow suicide?

Over the last 30 years or so, it seems that we have added nine times more sugar to our diet, according to statistics on its use. We have allowed a powerful new poison to invade our diet, it makes holes in the teeth and in the bones. Particularly saddening is the threat it poses to children's teeth. Adding fluoride to the water to protect teeth is avoiding the issue. The minute one eats sugar it starts of a reaction. The bacteria in the plaque on the teeth use sugar to produce an acid which attacks the enamel and the constant invasion of sugar will thus exacerbate dental problems. It is an empty food and only contains calories. It used to be thought that sugar was required for energy, but this is not the case. Sugar may well give us an increase in energy but that sudden burst will be short-lived. Sugar also, of course, brings about weight problems. Take my advice and read the labels when shopping for food. Sugar is widely used as a preservative, but watch out for glucose, fructose, maltose, dextrose and all similar additives in packaged and processed foods. For a safer natural preservative consider honey, raw cane sugar, molasses or muscavado, which at least are all less harmful forms of sugar.

Sugar is addictive and the source of endless problems. In my book *Realistic Weight Control*, I have advised how to reduce one's dependency on this substance and minimise its detrimental health effects. Count the many spoonfuls taken in tea or coffee, soft drinks, ice creams, jams, chocolates, etc. in a single day. Many people declare that they very soon feel better as they cut down on sugar and sugary foods like biscuits and cakes. Ironically, I have just noticed an advertisement promoting the sale of healthy ice cream. How can an ice cream be healthy if we think of the enormous amount of sugar it contains? The more luxurious and expensive the ice cream, the higher it is in saturated fats and calories.

Cutting down on sugar will be no problem, says the sugar addict, because I'll use an artificial sweetener. But here again we must be careful because artificial sweeteners are not always safe. They may be an enemy instead of a blessing for those with a sweet tooth. The great 'E-numbers' controversy has given us much to think about. There is a risk attached to the use of artificial sweeteners. Saccharine has been in use for over a century, yet its safety has never been proven and it has only provisionally been accepted. The cyclamates have caused great concern, especially in the UK, USA and Canada, and so I would stress that users of artificial sweeteners consider their addiction seriously and take action to reduce this dependency. Nature is a great provider if only we try to keep our food natural instead of introducing all these artificial additives and pampering our taste buds and cravings without regard for the effects on our health.

In a magazine I read that in the US alone 30,000,000,000 tins of food are sold each year. If we thought about how much sugar and salt is added to the food in these tins, would we still doubt that we serve up danger on a plate? It is no wonder that twentieth-century diseases are on the increase, some of which don't even have a name. Even if our only consumption of sugar is as a preservative, we are far from safe. At one time there was an outbreak of salmonella among a group of elderly people. Immediately it was claimed that the correct means of preservation of the suspect food had been used. Yet a salmonella virus had still been present, and that is the hidden danger. Cocci, staphylococci and streptococci are all increasing and I doubt if the preservatives in convenience foods are all they are claimed to be.

One of the greatest nutritional experts and lecturers in the world, Professor Arnold Ehret, said that 'life is a tragedy of nutrition. Man digs his grave with his knife and fork and we ought to give our body and our stomach a little rest.' Therefore occasional fasting, reduced intake of calories, carbohydrates, proteins and fats, without restricting vitamins, minerals or fibre, is a healthy practice and will lead to a healthier and more vital life. One fasting day a week will get rid of many of our toxins and will help the body to do its allotted task. Healing is within oneself.

Vinegar is yet another preservative, and as people get more and more hooked on savoury foods, its role as a preservative is on the increase. Because of the lack of potassium in the daily diet, it would be far better to use cider vinegar. This is a rich source of potassium and is an excellent alternative to malt and other kinds of vinegar. These products should not, however, be used on too regular a basis.

The Ministry of Agriculture, Fisheries and Food has published a book called *Food – Portions and Sizes*. The writer, Helen Crawley, gives us some indication of the amount of food we eat, by examining the weight of each food product. The same ministry has also published a good leaflet on food additives and, taken together with the book written on additives by Maurice Hansen, we must come to the conclusion that between them, preservatives and additives add up to a lot of trouble. Why not, for example, use Molkosan, which is a whey product, in a salad dressing instead of vinegar? Indeed, vinegar is often at the root of liver disorders, and it can affect the enzyme secretion in the stomach. A burning sensation will occur when there is an excessive gastric secretion. Vinegar can do a lot of harm, but by using Molkosan, which has a nicer flavour, we can improve our health.

All these preservatives destroy the living factors in food. We want to look for ways to increase energy, not deplete it. Friendly bacteria, which are needed, are simply killed off by such preservatives and this becomes apparent in bacterial imbalances. The digestive process can thus become impaired, sometimes causing acute distress. This brings me to the third health enemy in the group of the three S's and that is STRESS.

Stress is no respecter of sex, age, colour or creed, and strikes when circumstances allow. In my book *Stress and Nervous Disorders*, I have written about possible ways to avoid or reduce stress. One should understand that stress often occurs because of the wrong dietary management. It is easier to try and put the blame on the demands placed upon us every day by problems at work, resentment, jealousy, family arguments, financial stress, or deadlines to meet. But the stress factor is mostly caused by a disturbance of the balance of the body, mentally or physically. Many stress symptoms are in fact self-induced and relate to the way we look after ourselves and our health. This is why it is important to treat the subject in a book on food, where it can be approached from a different angle. A well-balanced diet will help to foster a balanced mental attitude.

Earlier in this chapter I pointed out the dangers of salt. In the same way that the adrenals are forced into distress because of the use of too much salt, so sugar affects the seven endocrine glands, which are responsible for good hormonal housekeeping. Naturally the body, when it is being attacked by these substances, sends out alarm signals and these mean stress. The heart rate goes up, the rate of the breathing increases, digestive secretions are reduced, blood sugar levels rise, and hypertension occurs. The body tells us, in its own language, that it is under stress and needs help. It's hardly any good swallowing a pill to reduce this stress if we are not interested in the underlying cause. The alarm bells are ringing, and they will not be stopped unless we correct the cause of the alarm. Nutritional management may need to be revised, so that the body receives the vitamins, minerals and trace elements it needs. If these are lacking in our food, we can introduce them by way of a supplement. Remember that there are many homoeopathic remedies that can be taken to reduce stress, and these will serve the person concerned much better than swallowing a tranquilliser.

Number one remedy is the daily diet. Because of stress and wrong dietary management, rheumatism and arthritis are an ever-growing problem. Stress is the biggest defaulter of potassium, which is so essential to arthritic people. With any sign of stress the tiny gland at the base of the brain, called the pituitary gland, releases a hormone into the bloodstream to reach the two small glands that sit on our kidneys in the middle of the back, the adrenals. When the adrenals pick up this hormonal messenger, they too will release hormones – the chief of these is called cortisol, better known as cortisone. Messages come from the nervous system too and the adrenalin hormone is also released. The presence of these adrenal hormones in the blood signifies that the whole body is under stress. During this process, the level of potassium, which is immediately endangered by stress and which acts as a secondary agent in this process, is reduced. The role of nutritional management and natural remedies is to support this stress situation and to allow a more healthy lifestyle. We must watch out for and correctly interpret such symptoms, as these are the body's way of telling us that it is in need of support. This language can only be understood if we pay careful attention. Do we have sudden bouts of irritability? Do we need tranquillisers or sleeping tablets? Do we lack interest in life in general? Do we crave more coffee than usual?

Do we try to do too much at once? Do we experience a feeling of stiffness when awakening in the morning? Does it take all our effort to get out of bed in the morning to face another day? These signs and many more indicate the presence of stress. We must learn to relax, both in our work and in our spare time. Decide on some form of exercise and reduce your food intake. Let your motto be: Eat to live and do not live to eat. Breathe in fresh air and work towards better physical fitness. Who wants to be overweight? Exercise the muscles and keep the vital organs in good order so that you can enjoy life to the full. Our body is our responsibility. Treat it well and it will stand you in good stead. How good it is to look in the mirror and to like what we see. It's well worth it.

13

Food Irradiation

IT MUST BE about 25 years ago that I attended a fascinating seminar in London on a topic which at that time had received only little attention. One of the most interesting people at the seminar was an American lady who spoke on the subject of food combining, although that term wasn't used in those days. She was an elderly lady whom I greatly respected for the ideas she expressed. Her name was Dr Hazel Parcells, and her knowledge about electromagnetic energy in food was greatly appreciated. She is a lady who practises what she preaches. She is now well past the age of 100 and still lectures occasionally, helping people to regain life, not to destroy it.

The ideas expressed at this seminar led to a concern on my part regarding food irradiation. It is a doubtful preservation technique which is used on certain food supplies which are probably already unsafe. Most definitely it cannot increase the quality of food and certainly irradiated food has no place in a healthy diet. As far as I am concerned, food irradiation is a health hazard and although it is usually done to kill poisonous bacteria, the electromagnetic energy which becomes present, and on which Dr Hazel Parcells spoke with such authority and expertise, renders the food of no value whatsoever. I assert that dangerous foods, that are being given an extended shelf life, contain no vitamins and no life. We live in times in which we need cell renewers, as there are plenty of cell breakers. We need 'lively' food. We need food that heals and not food that kills.

We should try with every means within our power to prevent the process of food irradiation becoming a normal practice, because once that is the case the process will be very difficult to stop, let alone reverse. Food irradiation must not be allowed. One reason is that there is, in fact, no effective test to discover if food has been irradiated. Only by enforcement of the law will we be able to protect ourselves against these practices. It is very regrettable that some countries have allowed it to become legal. Although there have been many complaints and objections, they have been unsuccessful. Britain has joined France and the Netherlands in allowing selected foods to be irradiated to ensure longer shelf life. However, in Germany the authorities have opposed this practice from the very beginning. In Britain, it is true, only certain foods are allowed to be subjected to irradiation treatment, but these foods are very much the ones that are supposed to give us life energy. In a special report written by Caroline Wheater in *Here's Health* of June 1991, we read that the dose of ionising radiation used – ranging from 1 to 10 kilorays – is equivalent in strength to between 10 and 100 million X-rays. To my great horror I read in her report that the first products likely to be irradiated will be herbs and spices, but that the law leaves plenty of room for other foods to be irradiated if and when manufacturers and producers wish to do so. She continues by saying that:

> Food irradiation is claimed to prevent breeding in fruits and grains, to inhibit the sprouting of vegetables, delay the ripening of fruits, and kill bacteria which can cause food poisoning, such as listeria, salmonella and

campylobacter. Supporters of irradiation say that less produce will be spoilt, the shelf life will be extended by around five days and food poisoning will be wiped out. Evidence to the contrary disturbs the anti-irradiation lobby which claims that the process is a licence to serve up bad food.

I often wonder if those who make decisions affecting other people's health know what life is all about. Until the nineteenth century we had very little nutritional knowledge. Now we know that life is a constant renewal of cells and that degenerative disease is the relentless breakdown of this renewal process. We also know that life is a chemical process and that the chemicals involved in this process are the chemicals contained in our food and drink. In principle we are a living form of the chemicals we retain from what we eat and drink. The connection between us and the food we eat could hardly be more intimate. We need life and body builders and not body breakers, which to me are what food irradiation brings about.

I managed to obtain a copy of a book published by the World Health Organisation in collaboration with the Food and Agricultural Organisation of the United Nations. In this book only slight reference is made to problems surrounding food irradiation. The authors try hard to convince us that the practice of food irradiation is totally acceptable and completely safe. Yet considering the heat treatment with which some fruit will be processed, one must wonder if there will be any life left when 'preservation' processes are finished. I believe that food is an integral part of the treatment of patients and the more 'lively' the food and the closer it is to its natural form, the better it deserves the name of life builder. This is something that Dr Hazel Parcells stresses continuously n her book *The Electromagnetic Energy in Food*. Food processing of any kind is a very complex subject: packaging and freezing etc. must all be watched very carefully. And in the WHO book we read that the technique and the equipment employed to irradiate food must pass all tests according to Health and Safety requirements although, due to the variety of problems that are unique to this way of processing, food irradiation must be seen in a category all by itself. Food irradiation is a particular form of applying electromagnetic energy, an energy of ionising radiation. X-rays as a form of radiation do indeed kill bacteria. However, in destroying bad bacteria the good bacteria suffer equally. Certainly the process will kill the energy in food which is essential to our diet.

Some studies have demonstrated that radiation often softens food, especially fruits. This allows the possibility that some of these fruits will develop an undesirable flavour. With high energy levels, ionising radiation can even make certain foods radioactive. I could be assured 100 times that those with the necessary expertise on the wholesomeness of irradiated food have come to scientifically safe conclusions concerning irradiated products and have caused all necessary precautions to be taken, but still I would be very concerned about this process. Unless it were absolutely necessary, I would fight against any form of food radiation. Anyone with any common sense must realise that any food processed in such a way can only lose its nutrients – its vitamins, minerals and trace elements. It is of little use to see apparently healthy and attractive food on display in the shops if its nutritional value has been destroyed. The human body is designed to process, digest and absorb fruits and vegetables in as fresh a condition as possible. That is when maximum benefit will be gained.

The WHO book also states that:

> The consequence of processing by irradiation is
>
> (a) the opportunity to treat foods after packaging to prevent microbes penetrating from contaminated food that has already been processed;
>
> (b) the conservation of food in a fresh state for long periods with no noticeable loss of quality;

(c) the economic savings from the use of a low energy,
low cost processing technique when compared with other
food processing methods, such as heat or refrigeration.

Put rather nicely, but this does not alter the fact that food irradiation is a totally unnatural method of preservation and cannot possibly enhance the quality of our food. We would do well to remember that life is all about the renewal of cells; food irradiation leaves one wondering what effect such a preservation process could have on the immune system. If we do not obtain the correct chemicals or nutrients from our food to allow our bodies to continue with the function of producing adequate supplies of the multitude of different cells, we cannot expect to remain in good health. Food that has been irradiated with rays similar to those used for taking X-ray pictures cannot fail to leave the nutrients sterile and lacking in all goodness. Although we are assured that food irradiated under the correct conditions does not become radioactive, from the homoeopathic point of view the procedure is quite possibly harmful.

Imagine 100 patents with similar symptoms. Because each individual is different, each of these 100 people would benefit from individual treatment and dietary recommendations. It has been said that food irradiation has been thoroughly tested over the last 30 years, but that a number of these tests produced inconclusive results. It would be very unfortunate to belong to the small group that is not quite sure what effects irradiation may have on food.

Irradiated food contains mutagens which, it is said, will not be destroyed. It is also stated that not every micro-organism is destroyed. The final responsibility lies with the consumer, who must see to it that appropriate precautions are taken with such food, such as refrigeration and correct preparation methods. People may be fooled with the statement that it is all quite safe. My sincere hope is that the consumer will check what he buys, and if the symbol indicating that the food has been treated with ionising radiation is seen, he will score that food off his shopping list. I would certainly refuse to eat it. Although the method has been approved in many countries, it worries me to think of the possible effects it may have in relation to the immune system. To my way of thinking irradiated foods can never be considered of any help to a failing immune system.

I spent some time in Australia not long ago where I praised their good sense in opposing the use of insecticides, an occurrence which was well publicised during one of my previous visits. Now I have learned that Australia has refused to allow the irradiation of food. I am happy indeed that the authorities in Australia, New Zealand and Germany are prepared to ban food irradiation. This, to me, is common sense. The public cannot be fobbed off with the simple statement that it is safe, unless there is sufficient evidence to back up such a statement. It is only logical that when the bad parts of food are destroyed the good ones will also be affected. Untreated food will begin to smell when it loses its freshness. To use an irradiation process to prevent the development of a smell that is supposed to warn us when food is deteriorating cannot stop that food from rotting at the allotted time in the body. The kind of food that has been irradiated is the type we need to keep 'alive' to maintain our energy and this is particularly worrying.

It is intriguing to learn that when sprouting seeds are irradiated to kill the larvae fly, these seeds will never sprout again as all life has been killed within them. Potatoes, which are a high quality food product, are sometimes subject to irradiation, to prevent sprouting in storage. It is also worth knowing that after irradiation these potatoes are known to be much more susceptible to fungus and the loss of irradiated potatoes is much greater than was anticipated.

It may be true that irradiation does not contaminate food nor make it radioactive, but irradiation takes place inside well-insulated, or pre-packaged, food, and it's anyone's guess what really happens to it. Purposely eliminating the nutritional value of our food and rendering it 'useless' for the purposes for which it was designed is something I'll never be able to condone. Thus I am delighted to see that some major firms in the food industry will not allow such a process to take place on their premises. I cannot stress sufficiently that we need food that heals and not food that kills. I agree with freedom of choice but it is important that decisions made in the best interests of mankind should be taken into account in their context.

The word irradiation alone sounds scary and recalls frightful memories, such as Hiroshima and Chernobyl, and the resultant dreadful cancer statistics. I cannot state for certain that irradiated food will cause cancer. I do say, however, that most likely it will influence the body cells in a detrimental fashion.

Cancer resembles warfare. Two armies are fighting: the army of degenerative cells against the army of regenerative cells. The more we can do to encourage and strengthen the regenerative cells the better, and I am very sceptical that this ongoing battle can be won by eating food that has been irradiated.

We all need to eat to live and we must eat the right food. I can only feel sorry for children who are given food without having any choice or control. This is the responsibility of the parents and they will be deciding the child's future. We agree that we need food with less additives and colourings and yet we tend to ignore the effects of food irradiation.

It has been questioned whether sufficient tests on food irradiation have taken place, but experiments have gone on for decades. The end result is still that nobody is completely sure as to its dangers. One cannot deny that radiation affects the energy transfer and almost certainly it will also change the structure of the food. We must do everything possible to keep the valuable immune properties in our vegetables, fruit and grains that nature has provided.

After the Chernobyl disaster German scientists carried out tests on food that had been grown organically and food that had been grown in the accepted commercial manner. Radiation tests are measured on the Geiger scale and if this reading exceeds nine we have reason to be worried. Both foods grown in the organic manner registered below 11, while some of those grown in soil with chemical additives topped a reading of 37. The conclusion here must be that organically grown foods have better immunity and by eating such food this immunity is transferred to the physical system of the consumer. It assists us in withstanding atmospheric attacks on our health. Commercially or 'artificially' grown food, as I sometimes call it, does not posses that immunity.

Surely it's better to have quality than quantity and if the quality of our food is of a high standard, the quality of life will be too. As Dr Hazel Parcells says, food that has electromagnetic energy is food that produces cells or cell tissue. Acid food (positive) and alkaline food (negative), if blended will create a neutral balance. That balance must be maintained and in the process our food must be kept clear of strong invaders. Allow nature to have its way and keep all food as natural as possible. Buy food that is in season. Try also to get food locally and, where possible, look for organically grown food. Look at the labels of any packaged foodstuffs and most especially I would ask you to check if the irradiation symbol can be found on the packaging. It is not difficult to recognise the quality of fruit or vegetables; it is obvious if they are fresh or in a state of deterioration. This obvious evidence will show the life in our food.

14

Fasting – Detoxifying Diets

AS PART OF my research work I visit British prisons, where I have interviewed a number of hardened criminals, some of whom are serving life sentences. During my work on this project I have learnt to look at food from various different angles. I have also learnt much about allergies and have written in depth on this subject in my book *Viruses, Allergies and the Immune System*. Every prison visit has involved and clarified different aspects of prisoners' behaviour. A while ago I was introduced to a prisoner who had decided to go on a hunger strike. This was his way of showing that he disagreed with his sentence. He refused to take any solid food and would drink only water. The interesting result of this was that the three allergies he used to suffer from cleared up completely. This is an obvious indication that allergy problems are often caused by eating the wrong food.

Fasting is a well-established and long-practised part of natural medicine. By fasting it is possible to get rid of an allergy, and it is also an extremely effective method of detoxifying the body. When fasting, the body disposes of waste material that has remained within it far too long. Fasting, however, requires a good deal of common sense as it is possible to misjudge the situation. This is sometimes seen in teenagers when it becomes Anorexia Nervosa. To put it simply, fasting is a wonderful way to give the body a rest. It should be done voluntarily for a predetermined period, whether this be a day, a week, or longer. When I look at people who, probably quite unnecessarily, have fasted for months, it is amazing how well the body is able to cope without adequate food and how few demands it makes. Most therapeutic fasts, however, are recommended for shorter periods, usually from one day to a week maximum and involve drinking water, mineral water or fresh juices.

In the clinic where Alfred Vogel and I worked together, Saturday was always a fasting day. The patients enjoyed it and had a day of rest. Only fruit juices were served at mealtimes. They were happy to lose weight, but even more, they felt very alert the day after and often suggested that they fast for longer periods. This actually does the body no harm at all. It is no good starving to death when suffering from hunger. Fasting should be voluntary. Very often it serves as a stimulant for the body by detoxifying and restoring it to its normal condition. Problems with the respiratory system and gastro-intestinal problems often disappear after a day of fasting. It is possible to fast for longer periods, but it is not advisable to do this too often, and only ever when under strict medical supervision. Although the body can survive without food for a long time, it should not become too used to it, because one easily loses perspective. For many stomach problems fasting can be helpful and in these circumstances raw juices are excellent. Raw potato juice, for example, can be taken during the day when fasting, alternately with cabbage juice and condensed bilberry and liquorice juice. Alfred Vogel advises thickened juices to be taken daily in doses from one half to three-quarters of an ounce. These should be kept in the mouth for a minute to ensure proper salivation – this will hasten the curative effect. To rid the body of much harmful waste material one should fast at regular intervals for a full day on fruit juices only. You might find the following information on suitable juices from a popular German fasting course useful:

Raw Juices

Fresh pressed apple, grape or carrot juice is like nectar from the gods compared to the bottled variety you can buy. Raw juices have remarkable healing properties. They form the basis of what we think is the best contribution the Germans ever made to renewing vitality and good looks. It's called the Rohsaefte-Kur and many Western Europeans use it to revitalise themselves after a long winter when people eat too much, exercise too little and spend far too many hours in heated offices and houses. We use it when we are feeling 'dead' from too much stress, too little sleep or just simple fatigue. The Rohsaefte-Kur is simply a raw juice regime which should be carried out over several days to spring clean the system and make you feel super-alive – mentally clear and wonderfully receptive to things around you. It makes the skin glow and also trims away a few excess pounds.

Raw juices are exceptionally rich in health-producing enzymes as well as vitamins, minerals and trace elements useful in restoring biochemical balance to the body. According to authorities on the Rohsaefte-Kur, raw vegetable and fruit juices accelerate the burning up and the elimination of accumulated wastes. This is why a day or two on juices is the cornerstone of a rejuvenation treatment at many expensive European health resorts.

Raw juices cannot be made in a food processor or blender. They require a special juice extractor – usually a centrifuge of some kind, into which you feed the fruits and vegetables as it chops them and spins out their precious juices. Then you are left with the juice which you drink and the pulp which you toss into the compost. The health–promoting properties of fresh juices depend on their being drunk alive – that is, within a few minutes of being made – so that the oxidation process which sets in almost immediately does not destroy essential vitamins and enzymes. We find, however, that if you make a Thermos full of juice and chill it immediately by filling it with ice cubes, it will keep for several hours, so you can take it to work or drink it throughout the day, when you feel thirsty.

Raw juices are by no means only valuable because of their therapeutic properties. Some – such as fresh apple, grape and pineapple – are also the best-tasting drinks available.

As part of a fruit juice fast, if it is necessary to thoroughly empty the bowels, Linseed or Linoforce are efficient laxatives. In more stubborn cases a chamomile enema is beneficial. By this method one rids the body of much waste material, so that the organs in the body will function better. If you feel unwell during a fast, a cold friction bath will speed up the elimination. Exercises for the circulation or deep breathing exercises will also help. It is amazing how clear the mind becomes after fasting, and it is said that Mahatma Gandhi made his best decisions during fasts.

In the case of a liver disorder, Alfred Vogel advises vegetable juices in preference to fruit juices. Carrot and beetroot juices are ideal.

The Schroth cure is a regime that helps to promote elimination and is very good for the stomach and for many minor health problems. A three-day cure, it is widely used.

First day

Eat dry toast before noon. Midday meal consists of oatmeal or rice porridge. From 4.00 p.m. dry wine or apple juice, rice or barley gruel. Cold pack at night.

Second day

Toast or dry biscuits before noon. Porridge with apple sauce for midday meal. After 4.00 p.m. herb tea, fruit juice or wine. Cold pack.

Third day

Toast, dried prunes, baked or jacket potato and lemon slices when thirsty.

Our domestic pets can teach us a lesson. When they are ill, they often refuse any food and it is surprising how long they can keep up such a fast. They usually do not start eating until they are on the mend. They will go without food and drink until their bodies have recovered.

The following example of the benefit of fasting is upsetting, but nonetheless true. Involuntary fasting took place in concentration camps and prison camps during the war, and yet many who suffered the indignities and starvation agree that it left them with a clear mind and full of determination to survive. I remember when my father returned from a concentration camp after the war. Considering how badly starved he had been and how emaciated he looked, he still had considerable mental strength.

A brief fasting regime is very beneficial for patients with *Candida albicans*, ME and other food-related problems. A short, sensible fast with fruit juices or vegetables promotes energy and quickly rebuilds the body.

In cases of *Candida albicans* and ME I have seen tremendous improvements when patients have used Alfred Vogel's Detox Box.

Frangula Complex. Take two to four tablets every morning and evening. Digestion will be improved due to the stimulation of the intestinal glands. If two tablets do not appear to be sufficient, the dose can be increased to three or even four. No more should be necessary. One tablet should suffice for children, to be taken with fluid. It is worth knowing that this formula is not addictive, [and] even when used for a long period of time, the results will still be successful as long as food intake is sensible.

Milk Thistle Complex. This is a fantastic remedy for an overworked, hung-over liver, struggling with the toxic burden placed upon it daily. Indications that the liver is not in peak condition are bad periods, bad skin, a metallic taste in the mouth, unfair weight gain especially around the abdomen, lethargy, problems with temperature regulation, and anaemia. As well as Milk Thistle, the tincture contains Dandelion root, Globe Artichoke, Peppermint and Boldo. Pop 15 to 20 drops into a little water twice a day.

Solidago Complex. Like Milk Thistle Complex this remedy was a great favourite with Alfred Vogel, and is a tonic for the kidneys. If your diet revolves around crisps, chocolate, coffee and fizzy drinks, you may well feel some kidney symptoms, such as puffy bags under the eyes in the morning, lower back pain, swollen fingers or ankles, thinning hair and fatigue. You may also get panic-attack-type symptoms due to dehydration. This Complex contains Golden Rod (Solidago), Birch, Restharrow and Horsetail. Taken twice a day in a little water, 10 to 15 drops of this tincture will help tone up your kidneys.

Calendula Complex. This remedy contains Calendula (Marigold), Viola Tricolor (Wild Pansy) and Echinacea purpurea. It is for the lymphatic system. It often improves adult acne and bad periods into the bargain. Remember that the lymphatic system works best if you manage to get some sort of physical activity into your day. Take 10 to 20 drops of the tincture twice a day in a little water.

At least one course per annum to cleanse the system is recommended. For people suffering from persistently sluggish bowel function it may need to be increased to two or possibly even three courses per annum.

The use of Alfred Vogel's Golden Grass Tea is recommended as this does not force, but supports the kidneys. Some other brands of kidney tea tend to be rather harsh. Golden Grass Tea should be taken without sugar if possible. If sweetening is required, use honey. Taken over a long period of time Golden Grass Tea has a stimulating effect, and used in conjunction with the Detox Box is beneficial for general wellbeing.

In addition to a sensible diet, such as that outlined below, drink 1.5 litres of still water every day, as this helps to flush out the urinary tract.

Breakfast
Oatmeal, bran flakes, or muesli cereal with cooked prunes and their juice
Natural yoghurt with honey
Toasted whole grain bread
Fresh fruit juice
Herb tea or Swiss Coffee Substitute

Lunch
Homemade vegetable soup (use Plantaforce bouillon and Herbamare or Herbamare Spicy for seasoning)
Rice or soya dishes with vegetables
Salad of your choice
Herb tea or Swiss Coffee Substitute

Dinner
Vegetables
Rice or potatoes
Salad of your choice (try using cider vinegar or Molkosan mixed with sunflower oil as a dressing)
Nuts or food with nuts
Yoghurt or cottage cheese

Herb tea or Swiss Coffee Substitute

Foods to Avoid

Pork, white flour, white sugar, butter, chocolate, alcohol, coffee and black tea. If you have *Candida albicans*, also avoid mushrooms, yeast products, cheese, salt and spices.

Special note

Do not use fruit and vegetables at the same meal. Use minimal seasoning and spices. While a vegetarian diet is recommended, fresh fish and poultry are preferable to red meat.

Another method of regular bowel cleansing is by eating unprocessed bran. A good tablespoonful of bran once or twice a day will result in a thorough cleansing. This is especially beneficial for problems such as diverticulitis and colitis.

Reasons for fasting should be looked at carefully. Illness can be divided into two categories: acute and chronic. It is easy for an acute illness to develop into a chronic illness, therefore protection is better than cure. Always consider the importance of the bowel bacteria and take care not to destroy them with drugs and antibiotics. Friendly bowel bacteria should be kept alive and even during a period of fasting, plain and natural food will maintain the strength of the patient. Three or four days on grapes or fruit juices may be helpful. This can be followed by a course of rice or sprouted wheat. This has been widely recommended by Dr Kristina Nolai and Dr Bircher Benner, who were great pioneers of fasting and diets.

During my last visit to the USA, in nearly every health food shop I visited, I was asked about fruit juices. A television programme had been extolling the virtues of fruit juices and juice fasting. I am all in favour of this but let's not forget that we have teeth for chewing and grinding food, and we should not encourage a lazy digestive and bowel system by taking our food in the form of juice. Saying this, I must immediately reiterate that juice fasting is of great help. I believe in the principle that fasting is the oldest and most effective healing method known to man. I also agree that juice fasting is superior to traditional water fasting. At Stobhill General Hospital in Glasgow a 54-year-old woman with a very painful arthritic condition was kept on a liquid fast for 249 days and she lost 74 of her 262 lbs. Her arthritic pains disappeared completely. This is evidence of what can be achieved.

Fasting is a safe and effective method of cleansing, regenerating and rejuvenating the body. The length of each fast is the individual's decision but it should be monitored by a doctor or practitioner. Water fasts, although, as said, perhaps inferior to juice fasts in some ways, can however also achieve great results and in my book *Water Healer or Poison?* I have outlined how such a fast should be done on the basis of the Kneipp hydrotherapy method.

It is important to have plenty of rest during a fast. Initially, it is possible that one may feel a little tired or even nauseated and light-headed, but this will disappear as the body adjusts. Don't stay in bed when fasting. Get out and about and do gentle exercise. Enjoy the sun, go swimming or take a ride on a bicycle. A daily bath or water treatment can be helpful.

I am wary of drinking too many citrus fruit juices. It is better to use other juices as well. Excellent teas for drinking during fasts include peppermint, rosehip, chamomile, ginseng, and tea brewed from *Harpagophytum* (Devil's Claw root). Make sure that you don't overeat after a fast. Slowly reintroduce natural food, if possible additive-free wholesome food, and chew it well. It is advisable to take extra vitamins, minerals and trace elements during a fast, which will also help if you should feel hungry. Fasting teaches us respect and discipline and this will never go amiss. It is a tremendous stimulant to prove that one can overcome addictions to, for instance, sugar, salt, coffee, tea, or alcohol. It is a time of rest. It makes us realise that we not only love our bodies, but also our mind and spirit. This is the old homoeopathic principle laid down by the founder of homoeopathy, Samuel Hahnemann, to treat body, mind and spirit. Our mind and spirit are improved during fasting and there is a great deal of truth in the old German proverb: 'A full stomach does not like to think.'

I have just finished reading the book *The Miracle of Fasting*, written by Paul and Patricia Bragg. The book draws the reader's attention to many of the benefits of fasting and one particular expression is strikingly in accordance with one of Samuel Hahnemann's principles: they speak of the importance of 'conserving one's vital force'. Fasting is, of course, the key to this and the authors go on to describe its promotion of internal cleansing and purification and its clearing out of much of the waste material the body harbours. Illness is disharmony and sickness is the body telling us that we have internal problems and possibly toxic wastes and poisons. To restore the vital force, these need to be cleared. The life force within us, which gives us the ultimate strength required to enable us to do our daily duties, needs to be restored. After all, not only great masters fasted, but the Prince of Life, Jesus Christ, fasted for 40 days to concentrate his mind on the most important things of life.

Most of my patients with back and neck problems are treated osteopathically, but even here on many occasions fasting has helped. I remember an evening when I was lecturing in a small town. I had spoken on the subject of back and neck problems and during question time an elderly lady put up her hand. She told me that she was a retired nurse and asked if I agreed that many back problems were caused by a non-evacuated bowel. She had seen many long-term sufferers troubled with severe and persistent constipation problems. She was quite right.

We all ought to make a decision to fast, and then see it through. The physical improvement, along with the strengthening of character and the victory of mind over body will be a rich and deserved reward. Fasting is the natural way to get rid of unwanted and unhealthy waste.

Before starting a fast it is best to eat raw salads and fresh fruits for the last few days prior to the fast, and one should also drink plenty of water. During a fast the best possible opportunity to stop drinking tea, coffee and chocolate is provided, together with the opportunity of breaking the alcohol and smoking habit. It's quite wonderful how the body works and how gratefully it reacts to even the slightest effort we put in for an improvement in our health. But if insufficient fluid is received by the body, the secretions of the glands are cut, saliva dries up and the mucous membranes send out distress signals. We want to drink because we are thirsty. In its own language the body asks for what it needs. Of all the lubricants the most basic and essential is water. We cannot survive without water, and in my book on that subject you can read that 70 per cent of the human brain consists of water. Our body uses water all the time. It is impossible to digest food without fluid or water. It is needed to stimulate the gastric glands in the stomach and for the absorption of solids and the secretion of waste material. In conclusion, detoxification through fasting is becoming very necessary and will be the cornerstone of natural healing. I admire the wisdom in the well-known saying of Dr Howard Hay: 'The way to be well is to stop being sick.'

15

Conclusion

WHEN GOD DECIDED the time had come to populate the earth, he chose the best possible area for the earliest representatives of the human race – the Euphrates valley. This semi-tropical area boasted all the food necessary for good health. Fruits, nuts, seeds and vegetables are the best foods to be found in creation. In those early days man was able to pick whatever was required for sustenance, just by reaching out. Unfortunately, when the human race multiplied and spread out, the diet changed. Goat's milk and cow's milk were added to the diet and people became familiar with grains. By populating other areas, different environments were experienced and therefore different kinds of food were needed, especially for colder climates. It was then that man started to introduce certain kinds of meat into the diet.

In later centuries there was considerable imbalance in food – in India and China, for example, where, because of religious influence, certain foods were forbidden. Hence only the stronger members of a race would survive. It has always been a mistake to change a food pattern that is endemic to a country or nation. Sometimes a change in diet can be a pleasant experience and will do no harm. However, the diet designed for Indians, for example, is unsuitable for Westerners in the long term.

I remember meeting a world-renowned health and nutrition expert on one of my visits to India. I asked him for his opinion on improving the health of a nation, of realising the slogan of the World Health Organisation: 'Health for All by the Year 2000'. We agreed that this was absolutely impossible so long as we continue to export junk food such as chocolate bars and fizzy drinks to so-called primitive nations. Certainly, Eastern diets may not be detrimental to the health of the people who were born in those parts of the world, but such diets may not agree as readily with the digestion of Westerners. Man must bear in mind where he was born and where he wants to survive, and decide on a healthy diet that will afford him the energy he needs. Our health is our own responsibility, and therefore we must use common sense to consider what we eat and how we live. Is it not possible, when the first people on earth began to eat from 'the apple of knowledge', that they made the mistake of eating the wrong apple? There was a rich supply of vegetables and fruits, nuts and seeds, and yet it was that one apple they craved, because it was forbidden. It is that forbidden food we all too often choose. We must realise that we are no different to those first people on earth who were tempted by the forbidden fruit. When we know that something is not good for us, it seems to have more appeal. This is the problem with all that is forbidden; it is often so tempting. Let me point out that in exchange for discipline and self-respect we will receive health, and therefore will be able to lead a happier life.

Many of the modern forbidden fruits cause allergies, and it must be remembered that we should not allow ourselves to be influenced by the bad habits of our friends or neighbours. What is important is how we as individuals deal with the responsibility of maintaining our own health. Let me tell the coffee addicts among my readers that the danger of heart problems is increased five times by drinking coffee and that it is a major contributory factor for

Britain's 150,000 annual coronary victims. Research has established that drinking nine cups of coffee a day increases the cholesterol in the blood by 20 per cent. This is just one of the many irresponsible acts we impose on our own health by eating and drinking the wrong things.

Those guilty of excess fat intake in the diet are obviously unaware of the World Health Organisation recommendations. A 30 per cent intake of fat should be composed of the following: 10 per cent saturates, 10 per cent mono-unsaturates and 10 per cent essential polyunsaturates. I have already mentioned that a little dietary fat is necessary: the body is unable to manufacture certain polyunsaturated fats, which happen to be necessary for good health. A balanced approach should ensure that essential fatty acids derived from seed oils and fish oils should be present in the daily diet. The *Guardian* of Thursday, 13 April 1989, featured a good article entitled 'Eating is Believing'. The author stated that certain ingredients are necessary and certain fats can be good, if they are chosen wisely. It doesn't benefit our health if we are self-righteous. Our health is our own responsibility and fortunately a matter of free choice. But let us make a wise choice. The evidence is clear when we see people who have taken care of their diet, and at an elderly age are still enjoying good health.

A mother consulted me about her young child. She told me that she had visited many doctors, but no matter what she did, nothing seemed to stop the infant's colic. When I asked her if she breast-fed the baby, she told me that there hadn't been any problems until the baby was weaned. I wondered why she had introduced cow's milk. It was as simple as that, because the mother had herself diagnosed what was wrong with the baby. The colic was basically no more than an allergic reaction to cow's milk. We worked out an alternative, the baby's milk was changed and indeed the colic disappeared. Sometimes the answer is very simple indeed, and therefore more likely to be overlooked. Nature's secrets are hidden and it is up to man to discover them.

It is never an impossible task to discover these secrets if only we make the effort. I had another patient who, despite taking many drugs, could not reduce her cholesterol to an acceptable level. I suggested that every day she eat a handful of garlic. I have spoken and written about this natural remedy often, and it is nothing new. For centuries this has been in practice and there is no reason why it should not be effective nowadays.

Increased body weight caused by over-indulgence and minor problems can easily be overcome if we pay attention to proper dietary arrangements. One need not be discontented with one's diet and one should be able to eat the very best foods available. Deciding to choose healthier good is no punishment; in fact, quite the opposite, because on the whole it is tastier. Using the right nutritional ingredients in a diet of good quality carbohydrates, perhaps including garlic and olive oil, can be both healthy and satisfying. Try eating fresh fruit and vegetables every day. Fresh fish, particularly some of the oily varieties, contain many fatty acids which are needed by the body to manufacture prostaglandins. These can reduce the risk of heart attacks, strokes or blood clotting. With this information is there any reason why we should continue to endanger our lives?

The other morning, my first patient of the day was a very pleasant looking gentleman. I asked what was wrong because he looked rather unwell. Ruefully, he told me that it was the morning-after effect and it would wear off during the day. In other words he was suffering from a hangover. Is it wise to over-indulge in such substances when they make us sick and unfit for work? We risk our lives by not appreciating the existence of a link between alcohol and serious disease. Why not eat and drink the right things and experience the feeling of being on top of the world?

Is the right food still available, since so many fertilisers, pesticides, etc. are permitted in agriculture? I am in no doubt that the use of these substances causes our food to become more and more deficient in nutrients, minerals and trace elements.

But certainly, it is still possible to get wholesome fruit and vegetables and there is nothing to prevent you digging over a plot in the back garden and growing some of your own vegetables so that at least you know that the right organic manure has been used. Where there's a will, there's a way – remember, our body deserves the best possible supply of vitamins, minerals and trace elements.

Take care how you prepare and cook your food. Apart from using the right ingredients, make sure you use the right equipment. I know perfectly well when I have travelled by plane that the food I have been offered has been heated up in a microwave oven. That method of food preparation doesn't suit me and my body definitely lets me know that it is less than happy. Microwave cooking is an unnatural method of food preparation and destroys much of the vital force within the food. Eating industrially prepared food deprives us of many of the essentials and can easily lead to a premature degenerative process. The human body must be given the chance to defend itself against invaders and microbes, and our defence mechanism requires a higher level of immunity than ever before. This level of immunity is entirely dependent on how the body is treated. The most common agents of disease are bacteria, viruses and parasites. We have to defend ourselves against their attacks. A strong immune system, minimal toxins and a good diet, with adequate digestion, assimilation and elimination are effective allies to support us in any attacks on our health. Mathematics is not required, but common sense is. There is a right and a wrong way of eating and that applies to everyone. Most people eat the wrong food and this can be avoided simply by looking up a few nutritional details. Therefore, in summing up, I have made a list of a few foods, some that endanger our health and some that I have classed as relatively safe.

Danger Foods

Chocolate, cordials and fizzy drinks
White sugar and white flour
Cooked flour products
Fermented, processed, smoked and pickled foods
Cow's milk and cheese
Oranges and tomatoes
Tea and coffee
Pork in any shape or form
Fish oil (allergies only)
Malt vinegar
Refined salt
Excess animal protein and fats
Red wine

Relatively Safe Foods

Fresh fruit and vegetables
Soya milk and curds (Tofu)
Carob chocolate, honey, molasses and black sugar
Whole rye, rice, millet and buckwheat flour
Whole rye crispbreads
Whole grain rice, millet and buckwheat
Pulses and vegetable protein
Grapefruits, lemons and limes
Lamb, if meat is required, or white sea fish
Dandelion coffee, herb and China teas
Unsweetened fruit juices
Polyunsaturated vegetable oils
White wine
Cider vinegar
Sea salt

I advise everyone who has not previously taken notice of 'good' and 'bad' foods to start now. Slowly introduce substitutes, as it may be difficult for the body to cope with a drastic change. A gradual change is also a better incentive. It requires a great deal of discipline to break too many habits on the spur of the moment. Remind yourself of what is good and bad for you. The body will tell you what agrees and disagrees. With a little determination you will live up to the challenge and begin to feel more vital. Overweight people will soon feel slimmer and experience less obstruction, resulting in more energy.

A fresh approach to good health does not need to be in the form of a diet, although I have used this word for ease. The word diet is too often associated with a weight-reduction regime, but to me it primarily means more sensible eating, drinking and ensuring sufficient relaxation in our spare time. In that way one gains more self-respect, which in turn increases our determination to continue this new regime. In turn we learn to respect the food we eat.

I would also like to point out that it would do no harm to respect food more openly. The custom of asking a blessing on one's food should not be seen as old-fashioned. I prefer to see it as a thanksgiving for the food given by our Creator. The digestive process does not take kindly to a hurried meal. And when eating in front of the television, food isn't even tasted properly. Respect food as representing the necessary nutritional building blocks to keep the body in optimum health, and abide by the modern psychiatric and psychological view that eating should be a peaceful, relaxed and happy event. So many people, when under stress, attack and gulp their food, and don't even chew it properly. These people miss out on the wonderful opportunity to converse and relax during mealtimes and so heap more emotional stress upon themselves. Spare a moment at the beginning of the meal. A brief pause can be a mark of gratitude for food that blesses the body, the mind and the spirit. We are what we eat and what we drink. Too often the love and the labour expended in the preparation is totally ignored when the food is not eaten with a spirit of gratitude. The other day I watched in astonishment a lovely family in the dining-room of a hotel. They attacked their food without any visible sign of pleasure or gratitude and seemed intent on eating in the shortest possible time. No time even for a few polite remarks amongst themselves; they couldn't rush their meal quickly enough. Unfortunately, the parents were showing their children the worst example possible.

Our body is like a temple that serves us as well as other people. I read a beautiful saying by Henry David Thoreau:

> Every man is the builder of a temple called his body. We are all sculptors and painters and our material is our own flesh, blood and bones. Any nobleness begins at once to refine a man's features. Any meanness and sensuality to embrute them.

I could write much more about food, because it is a subject that is the essence of life. At lectures I am asked endless questions on food, food patterns, food management and food combining. Having answered such questions I always end by pointing out that the way to good health is to realise that the first rule of alternative medicine is sensible dietary management. We all rely on food, but let it be good food. Hippocrates said that 'the natural healing force within each one of us is the greatest force in getting well'.

Bibliography

Paul and Patricia Bragg, *The Miracle of Fasting*, Health Science, Santa Barbara, California, USA.

Deepak Chopra, *Creating Health*, Houghton Mifflin, Boston, USA

Helen Crawley, *Food Portion Sizes*, Thorsons, Hammersmith, London.

Department of Health, *Dietary Values for Food Energy*, HMSO Publishing.

Nigel Dudley, *Good Health on a Polluted Planet*, Thorsons, Hammersmith, London.

Robert Erdmann and Meirion Jones, *Fats, Nutrition and Health*, Thorsons, Wellingborough, England.

Elizabeth Evans, *Diet and Nutrition*, Octopus Books, London.

Doris Grant and Jean Joyce, *Food Combining for Health*, Thorsons, Hammersmith, London.

Dorothy Hall, *The Natural Health Book*, Thomas Nelson, Melbourne, Australia.

Maurice Hanssen, *E for Additives*, Guild Publishing, London.

Nicholaas Hartman, *De Natuurlijke Voeding voor de Mens*, De Driehoek, Amsterdam, The Netherlands.

Ross Horne, *The Health Revolution*, Ross Horne, NSW, Australia.

Ministry of Agriculture, *Food Hygiene*, HMSO Publishing.

Dugald Semple, *Home Cures for Common Ailments*.

A. Vogel, *Swiss Nature Doctor*, A. Vogel Verlag, Teufen, Switzerland.

Jan de Vries, *Traditional Home and Herbal Remedies*, Mainstream, Edinburgh, Scotland.

Tony Webb, Tim Lang and Kathleen Tucker, *Food Irradiation, Who Wants It?* Thorsons, Wellingborough, England.

World Health Organisation, *Food Irradiation*, WHO and Food and Agriculture Organisations of the United Nations.

Index